Anatomy, Stretching
& Training for Marathoners

Anatomy, Stretching & Training for Marathoners

A Step-by-Step Guide to Getting the Most from Your Running Workout

**Philip Striano, DC
and Lisa Purcell**

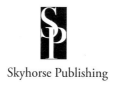

Skyhorse Publishing

CONTENTS

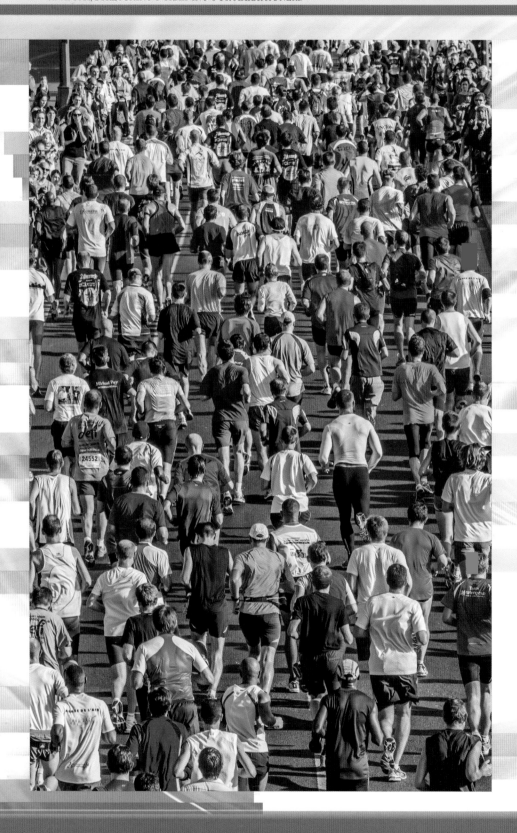

INTRODUCTION: WHY RUN A MARATHON?

Running and jogging are among the most popular recreational sports in the world. And thousands of competitors from around the globe sign up for marathons every year. So why do so many people from diverse backgrounds choose to run? Of course, each individual has unique motivations, but there are several goals shared by many runners, from a desire to lose weight to a need to lower blood pressure and strengthen the heart. From there, they develop a passion for running that takes them to the streets, whether a local competition or one of the big events, such as the London, Boston, Paris, or New York marathons.

Running is also a versatile way to get fit—you can run just about anytime and anywhere, and it is a relatively inexpensive sport. It doesn't require pricey health club memberships or personal training fees, and even the major marathons are still relatively affordable. With little more than the right pair of shoes, anyone of just about any age and fitness level can start a training program, and eventually run marathons.

Yet, as with any physical activity, there is a right way and a wrong way to run—don't expect to just lace up your running shoes and hit the pavement. You should also prepare for and augment your runs with stretches and exercises geared to warming you up before a run and cooling you down after it, and perform strengthening and stability exercises that target the key muscles used in running. Take the time to learn how to run right, using the guidelines found in the following pages, and you'll soon be entering that 26K.

RUNNING BASICS

MOST OF US ARE AWARE that running is a great way to lose weight and to get leaner and stronger, but its benefits are so much more than skin deep. Running is not just about improving your appearance. In fact, running is more about improving your overall health and allowing your body to perform at its highest levels. These are some of the most common reasons for running and the benefits you'll receive:

Burns calories

Running burns about 100 calories per hour (the more you weigh, the more calories you'll burn), so weight loss is a prime incentive for many beginner runners, and weight maintenance for those who run regularly.

Increases lean body mass

Your lean body mass is made up of everything in your body besides fat, including your organs, blood, skin, bones, and muscles. In general, a lower fat-to-muscle ratio is healthier.

A regular running regimen reduces fat and thereby lowers your fat-to-muscle ratio.

Increases VO$_2$ max

Your VO$_2$ max, or maximal oxygen consumption, is generally the amount of oxygen your body can transport and use during exercise that increases in intensity over time. Peak oxygen uptake equals peak physical condition—increasing your VO$_2$ max allows you to perform at your best.

Regulates cholesterol levels

Regular running can help you regulate cholesterol levels, lowering the "bad" LDL cholesterol levels, while increasing the "good" HDL levels.

Increases bone density

Since running is a weight-bearing exercise, it increases bone density—the measurement of the mineral content inside your bones. This helps protect you from osteoporosis-related fractures.

Improves your psychological health and self-esteem

The psychological benefits of running are many. With its endorphin-boosting power, running decreases stress and increases confidence. Running allows you to easily set—and meet—tangible goals, such as increasing your distances in less time during marathon training, which makes you feel good about yourself. It also improves your self-image; the physical changes you see in the mirror will give your self-esteem a boost and provide you with the incentive to stick to your training.

How to get started

Ease into a running routine. You want to incrementally build your strength and endurance; as your muscles and cardiovascular system adapt, you can slowly begin to build on your increased capacity. Taking it slow will help you prevent injury and avoid frustration.

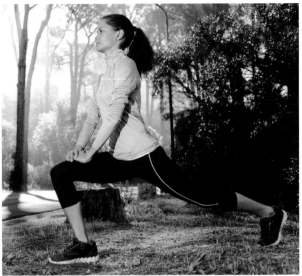

Before beginning any exercise regimen, check with your general practitioner to make sure that you are healthy enough to run and see whether you need to allow for any special considerations in your running routine.

Warming up and cooling down

To get the most from your run, take the time to warm up before you set out and cool down when you stop.

Proper stretching can lead to better performance, and you should make it a key component of both your pre-run warm-up routine and your post-run cool-down. Never stretch cold muscles, which are more prone to injury. To warm up before a pre-run stretch, take just 5 minutes to run in place, skip, or do a few push-ups—any activity that gets the heart pumping and blood flowing into muscles. After your run, again take a few minutes to perform some stretching exercises.

BORN TO RUN

Running may be one of the most natural forms of exercise you can choose. Scientific evidence suggests that the human body evolved quite literally to run—and to run over long distances. Our flexible leg and foot ligaments and tendons act like springs, and our narrow midsections allow us to swing our arms and keep us from weaving off a trail. A highly developed sense of balance keeps us stable while on the move. Even our toes are made for running—they are relatively short compared to our ape relatives', and our big toes are straight, which allows for a solid push-off from the ground. And the largest muscle in our bodies—the gluteus maximus—really only engages while we run. Numerous sweat glands and little body hair also make for a very efficient cooling system. So although we are no match for four-legged animals in a quick sprint, when it comes to covering long distances over many hours, few could keep up.

Take it slowly

If you are new to running, start by walking 20 minutes three times a week. Do not walk on consecutive days—allow your body to recover between walking sessions.

During the second week, if you feel fine physically, combine walking and running for 20 minutes on three non-consecutive days. Don't worry if you get tired—alternate running and walking at a pace that feels right for your body.

During the third week, jog or run for 20 minutes, again three times on non-consecutive days. If you need to pause, take a walking break, but don't stop. Keep yourself moving, and start running when you feel good again.

As the weeks pass, slowly increase the intensity, duration, and frequency of your running sessions, paying close attention to your body's response. If you overdo it, running too hard or too long or too often—ease back on your running schedule until you feel yourself getting stronger.

Remember—everyone's body is unique, so don't get frustrated if you are not getting immediate results. Find your own pace.

Dressing to run

No special clothing is required for running—just be sure to wear weather-appropriate attire (and avoid running at all during extreme weather, whether hot or freezing).

In warm weather, light-colored, loose-fitting clothing will help your

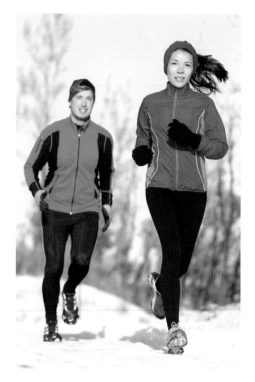

body breathe and cool itself naturally. Synthetic fabrics, which wick away moisture, are also better than natural cotton, which holds sweat. Sunglasses and a visor are also recommended to protect your eyes from any of the sun's harmful rays.

In cold weather, go for layers. Next to your skin wear synthetic or silk undergarments, such as long johns. Over that, add an insulating layer, such as fleece, and, over it all, add wind- and weatherproof outer garments. A neck warmer, bandanna, or balaclava can also protect your neck and face from the elements. And don't forget your hat—you lose much of your body heat through your head.

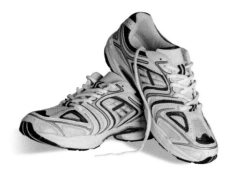

Running shoes

Running requires a proper pair of running shoes that support your feet and help to protect your body from injury. Choosing an appropriate pair starts with knowing your feet. You may think you know your size, but if possible have each foot measured at a reputable store that specializes in sports footwear. Determine your arch shape, which affects how you move or run. Are yours normal or high, or are you flat-footed? Going to a specialist running shop will help you determine if you over- or underpronate the foot.

TOO MUCH OF A GOOD THING?

Running makes you feel great, and turning it into a habit can do wonders for you physically and mentally. Marathoners must be committed runners, but some runners turn that habit into an addiction, pushing themselves to run ever farther, faster, and more frequently. Not only is this bad for them psychologically—they let family, friends, work, and community take second place to the need for additional running hours or run no matter how ill or fatigued—it also places them at risk for debilitating injury. Remember: even good things taken to the extreme can be bad for you.

All of these factors will help you choose the right kind of shoe for your unique way of running, whether ones that stabilize, cushion, or control motion. Once you've found the perfect shoes, don't just lace them on and go. Take the time to break them in gradually. And don't keep running in an old pair of shoes—most last between 300 to 400 miles.

Sports bras

For women, a comfortable bra is essential. The right running bra will work a delicate balance between adequate support and comfort. You want to find one that minimizes movement but doesn't constrict or bind. Look for one made of a moisture-wicking fabric that is relatively seam free to prevent chafing.

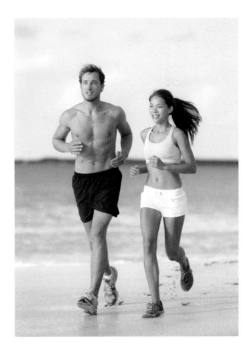

WHERE TO RUN

YOU CAN RUN just about anywhere, on just about any surface, from soft sand to hard concrete, but be aware that your body will react to the impact in different ways. Changing your running routine now and then is a smart plan—by switching between a variety of surfaces you can better strengthen muscles, ligaments, and tendons, and lower the risk of repetitive-strain injuries and muscle imbalances.

Grass

Close-cropped grass is one of the best surfaces upon which to run. It is a soft, low-impact surface that works your muscles hard, which will build strength, and flat grass is an excellent option for speed work. Grass does have its cons, though—it is often uneven and can pose danger for runners with weak

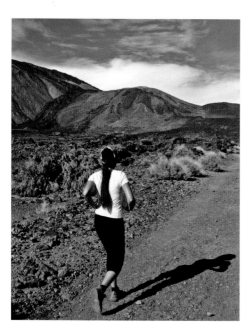

ankles. Longer grass may also hide hazards such as animal holes or rocks. Grass also turns slippery when wet, so if your regular routine takes you through grassland, plan an alternate route on rainy or damp days.

Woodland trails

Many parks and forests have woodland trails that seem designed for runners, with changing scenery that makes for an interesting run. Well-maintained, level trails of soft, well-drained peat or wood chips are easy on the legs, leading to well-rounded development of your muscles, ligaments, tendons, and joints. Not all trails are equal, though—without maintenance, these surfaces can deteriorate. In forests, tree roots or other debris may present tripping hazards, and in wet weather, trails can turn muddy and slippery.

Off road/dirt trails

This category covers quite a lot of ground, from rural roads to urban parks. Depending on where you live, the composition of dirt can range from dry, sandy soil to moist, clay earth. Most dry dirt surfaces will be medium to soft, which decreases your risk of injury from excessive training. It also reduces the impact of downhill running. Wet weather, unfortunately, turns a dirt trail into slippery mud. It is hard to run in mud, placing added stress on vulnerable areas such as calves and Achilles tendons and increasing your risk of injury.

Synthetic track

Outdoor tracks are ideal for speed work and interval training, with flat, forgiving surfaces and easy-to-measure distances. Yet many runners may find tracks less than exciting—it can get very boring very quickly to simply run in a circle. Running on a track may also increase your risk of injury. Those two long curves on every lap means you tend to land harder on the inside leg or pronate the foot, which can place extra stress on your ankles, knees, and hips.

Tarmac/asphalt

One of the most common road surfaces, tarmac (or asphalt) is also one of the fastest surfaces on which to run. At its best it is a predictable, even surface that places no added stress on your Achilles tendon; at its worst, it presents traffic, potholes, and a hard, unforgiving surface. Many tarmac roads are cambered or banked on the sides, which may cause you to run with an imbalanced stride that could lead to a foot, ankle, knee, hip, or muscle injury.

Sand

Like dirt, sand varies a great deal, from a flat, firmly packed surface to a loose, uneven one. Flat and firm is ideal, offering a forgiving, low-impact surface. Running on dunes provides good resistance training and a leg-strengthening workout. Running in soft sand will really work your calf muscles while going easy on your joints, but it does mean a higher

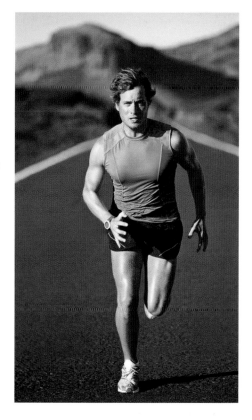

risk of Achilles tendon injury. Running on beach sand is also a very pleasant way to pass the time, with sea breezes and lovely shore scenery. Sand also gives you the opportunity to shed your shoes and run barefoot.

Concrete

Concrete may just be a fact of life for city runners—most pavements are made up of this cement-based surface. Its accessibility is its chief charm, but it is the surface hardest on a runner's legs. Add to that the hazards of curbs, pedestrians, and stop-and-go traffic lights, and this surface is less than ideal.

MARATHON TRAINING PRIMER

FINISHING A MARATHON is a feat few achieve, but with the right preparation you can join the ranks of those who cross the finish line. Just prepare yourself well, and give yourself adequate time to train properly.

Are you ready?

Your first question is not about how far you can run, but for how long. Can you run without stopping for at least 30 minutes? Next, have you been running for at least six months, logging distances of about 10 to 15 miles? If your answer is "yes" to these questions, you can begin a training regimen that will prepare your body for the challenge ahead. Of course, check with your doctor before undertaking any marathon training.

If you answered "no" to any of the above, work on a pre-training regimen—for absolute beginners, combine walking and running to get your body used to the demands a long-distance run places on it.

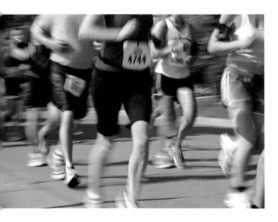

Make the commitment

Once you've determined that you are ready to begin training, be sure to set aside the time you'll need to fully prepare. Beginner runners and first-time marathoners planning to enter a 26.2-mile race typically need 20 weeks of training to get ready for race day.

As the sample training schedule (opposite) shows, preparing for a marathon involves a regimen of running, exercising, and resting.

Running

Plan to run every other day: Tuesday, Thursday, and Saturday, for example. After warming up, your Tuesday run should be at a moderate pace for the designated miles, only incrementally increasing your distances as the weeks pass. Your Thursday run is similar; run at a moderate pace, but gradually increase your distances by a bit more until the weeks right before the race.

Your Saturday run will be the real challenge: you need to add a mile or two each week. Keep a steady, easy pace for your Saturday run—you should be able to breathe easily and talk comfortably the entire time. As you get closer to the marathon, however, you need to reduce your distances. You want a rested and strong body on race day.

You can also add a Sunday run, but keep the distance short, and keep a slow, steady pace on easy terrain.

SAMPLE MARATHON TRAINING SCHEDULE

WEEK	MONDAY	TUESDAY	WEDNESDAY	THURSDAY	FRIDAY	SATURDAY	SUNDAY
1	rest	3-mile run	exercise	3-mile run	rest	4-mile run	3-mile run
2	rest	3-mile run	rest	3-mile run	exercise or rest	5-mile run	3-mile run
3	rest	3-mile run	exercise	4-mile run	exercise or rest	6-mile run	3-mile run
4	rest	3-mile run	rest	4-mile run	exercise or rest	4-mile run	3-mile run
5	rest	4-mile run	exercise	4-mile run	exercise or rest	6-mile run	3-mile run
6	rest	4-mile run	exercise	4-mile run	exercise or rest	8-mile run	3-mile run
7	rest	4-mile run	exercise	4-mile run	exercise or rest	10-mile run	3-mile run
8	rest	4-mile run	exercise	4-mile run	exercise or rest	8-mile run	3-mile run
9	rest	4-mile run	exercise	4-mile run	exercise or rest	12-mile run	rest
10	4-mile run	4-mile run	rest	4-mile run	exercise or rest	10-mile run	3-mile run
11	rest	4-mile run	exercise	4-mile run	exercise or rest	14-mile run	3-mile run
12	rest	5-mile run	exercise	5-mile run	exercise or rest	10-mile run	3-mile run
13	rest	4-mile run	exercise	5-mile run	exercise or rest	16-mile run	3-mile run
14	rest	4-mile run	exercise	5-mile run	exercise or rest	12-mile run	3-mile run
15	rest	4-mile run	exercise	5-mile run	exercise or rest	18-mile run	rest
16	3-mile run	5-mile run	rest	6-mile run	exercise or rest	12-mile run	3-mile run
17	rest	4-mile run	exercise	6-mile run	exercise or rest	20-mile run	3-mile run
18	rest	4-mile run	exercise	4-mile run	exercise or rest	12-mile run	3-mile run
19	rest	3-mile run	20-mile run	3-mile run	exercise or rest	8-mile run	3-mile run
20	rest	2-mile run	20-mile run	rest day	20 -mile	race day	rest day

Exercising

If you follow the Tuesday-Thursday-Saturday-Sunday running schedule, pencil in Wednesdays and Fridays as exercise days. This could be a cross-training activity, such as swimming or cycling, or one of the exercise workouts included in this book. If you are feeling sore, though, use this as another rest day.

Resting

Resting is as important as running and exercising. Allowing your body to recover is essential to successful training. Take notice of any pain or soreness, and use your rest days to take appropriate preventative action to avoid injuries that will take you out of race before you are even in it.

COMMON RUNNERS' INJURIES

ADOPTING A MARATHON training schedule has numerous physical benefits, but your joints and muscles can take a pounding, leaving them susceptible to injury. Learning to recognize and avoid common running injuries is essential to a successful running routine.

Pushing yourself too hard, past your unique limitations, is a major cause of many running injuries. Beginners may run too often or too far, before they have become fully conditioned, and advanced runners may begin to add distance or

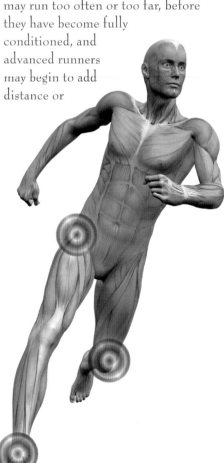

speed, tackle rougher terrain or run in any weather. Always keep in mind your particular body design, and adapt your expectations to account for your real strengths and weaknesses.

COMMON INJURIES

Your hips, knees, legs, and feet do most of the work of running and are therefore the body parts most vulnerable to injury. Here are some of the most common injuries runners face, their usual causes and symptoms, and the typical treatments for relieving them. Keep in mind that every individual may experience symptoms differently, but if you think you have sustained an injury, consult a doctor.

Runner's knee

A dull pain around the front of the knee (patella) where it connects with the lower end of the thigh bone (femur) is the primary symptom of runner's knee, also known as patellofemoral pain syndrome. It is commonly due to the kneecap being out of alignment. Its causes can be structural, such as a kneecap located too high in the knee joint, or induced, such as running with the feet rolling in, while the thigh muscles pull the kneecap outward.

Causes

• Structural defects
• Weak thigh muscles
• Tight hamstrings or Achilles tendons
• Improper foot support
• Improper form
• Excessive training or overuse

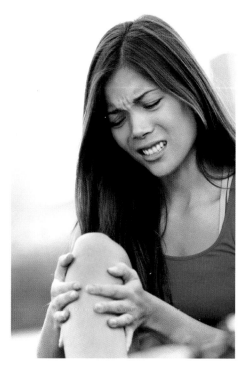

Symptoms

- Pain in and around the kneecap when going up or down stairs
- Pain in and around the kneecap when squatting
- Pain in and around the kneecap while sitting with the knee bent for a long time
- A feeling of knee weakness or instability
- Rubbing, grinding, or clicking sound when bending or straightening the knee
- Kneecap is tender to the touch

Treatment

- Cessation of running routine until injury is healed
- Cold packs, compression and elevation
- Pain-relief medication, such as ibuprofen
- Stretching exercises
- Strengthening exercises
- Adding arch support in shoes

Shin splint

Pain running along the front or inside of the shin bone (tibia) is a common runner's complaint. Many runners incur shin splints when they boost their running routine too quickly—adding too many miles or running too often without giving the body a chance to properly recover. Like runner's knee, the causes may be structural or induced. Shin splints involve damage to one of two groups of muscles along the shin bone. An anterolateral shin splint affects the front and outer part of the shin muscles and is caused by a structural imbalance in the size of opposite muscles. A posteromedial shin splint affects the back and inner part of the muscles of the shin. Any running can cause a posteromedial shin splint, as can running in improper shoes. People with flat feet are also prone to shin splints.

Causes

- Structural defects
- Improper foot support
- Excessive training or overuse

Symptoms

- Pain on the front and outside of the shin when the heel touches the ground while running that eventually becomes constant (anterolateral)
- Pain on the inside of the lower leg above the ankle that eventually becomes constant (posteromedial)
- Shin is painful to the touch (posteromedial)
- Pain when standing on the toes or rolling the ankle inwards (posteromedial)
- Inflammation (posteromedial)

Treatment

- Cessation of running routine until injury is healed
- Stretching exercises
- Strengthening exercises
- Cold packs
- Pain-relief medication, such as ibuprofen
- Wearing running shoes with a rigid heel
- Adding arch support in shoes
- Slow return to activity after several weeks of healing

PLANTAR FASCIITIS

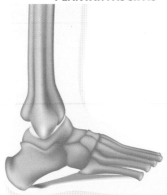

Inflammation of the plantar fascia

Plantar fasciitis

Plantar fasciitis is an inflammation of the thick band of tissue in the bottom of the foot that extends from the heel to the toes, called the plantar fascia. Plantar fasciitis produces severe pain in the heel, especially when you stand up after resting. If you are overweight, work in an occupation that requires a lot of walking or standing on hard surfaces, have flat feet, or have high arches, you may be susceptible to plantar fasciitis and should keep this in mind as you develop your training routine.

Causes

- Excessive training or overuse
- Tight calf muscles

Symptoms

- Severe pain in the heel of the foot

Treatment

- Rest
- Cold packs
- Nonsteroidal anti-inflammatory medications
- Stretching exercises

Stress fractures

Most often occurring in the lower leg or the foot, stress factures are tiny fissures in the surface of a bone. You are most likely to suffer from a stress fracture if you increase the intensity or frequency of your runs over several weeks or months or if your body is low in calcium. The tibia (the inner and larger bone of the leg below the knee), the femur (thigh bone), the sacrum

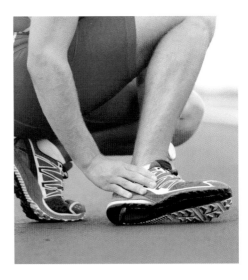

(the triangular bone at the base of the spine) and the metatarsal (toe) bones are the most susceptible to stress fractures. If you suspect that you have one, stop your running routine, and consult a physician as soon as possible—left untreated these tiny cracks can spread to become a full bone fracture.

Causes
- Excessive training or overuse
- Structural defects

Symptoms
- Muscle soreness that comes on gradually in the affected area
- Stiffness in the affected area
- Pinpoint pain on the affected bone

Treatment
- Cessation of running routine until injury is healed
- Rest
- Nonsteroidal anti-inflammatory medications
- Stretching exercises
- Muscle strengthening
- A cast or other form of immobilization of the area, depending on the severity of the injury
- Physical therapy (for severe fractures)

Iliotibial band syndrome

Iliotibial band syndrome, usually shortened to IT band syndrome or simply ITBS, affects the long ligament that runs along the outside of the thigh, from the top of the hip to the outside of the knee. ITBS occurs when this ligament thickens and rubs the knee bone, producing inflammation. Certain structural factors may make you more susceptible, such as a difference in length between one leg and the other. How you run and where you run also plays a role in the development of ITBS; for example, long-distance runners are more likely to develop ITBS.

Causes
- Tight or wide iliotibial band
- Weak hip muscles
- Overpronation of the feet
- Excessive training or overuse
- Excessive hill running
- Running on cambered surfaces
- Difference in leg length

Symptoms
- Pain occurring on the outside of the knee
- Tightness in the iliotibial band
- Pain aggravated by running, particularly downhill
- Pain during flexion or extension of the knee
- Weakness in hip abduction

Treatment
- Rest
- Avoiding painful stimuli, such as downhill running
- Cold packs after you run
- Decreasing the frequency, duration or intensity of your runs
- Heat and stretching prior to exercise
- Self-massage

ANKLE SPRAINS

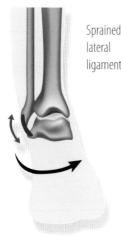
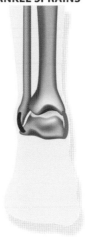

Sprained lateral ligament

Sprained medial ligament

INVERSION

NORMAL

EVERSION

Ankle sprain

An ankle sprain is the stretching or tearing of the ankle ligaments (the tough bands of elastic tissue that connect bones to one another). You are most likely to incur a sprain when your foot twists or rolls inward. The symptom and treatment of ankle sprains vary depending on the severity of the stretching or tearing.

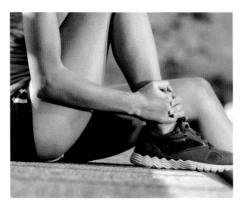

Causes

• Awkward foot placement
• Running or walking on irregular surfaces
• Weak muscles
• Loose ligaments
• Improper footwear

Symptoms

• Swelling
• Pain
• Bruising

Treatment

• Resting the ankle
• Wrapping the ankle with bandage or tape
• Cold packs
• Elevating the ankle
• Gradual return to walking and exercise
• A walking cast (for moderate sprains)
• Surgery (for severe sprains)
• Physical therapy (for severe sprains)

Achilles tendonitis

Runners often experience the effects of Achilles tendonitis. The Achilles tendon, running from the heel to lower calf, is the largest and most vulnerable tendon in the body and joins the gastrocnemius and the soleus muscles of the lower leg to the heel of the foot. Although the Achilles tendon is strong, it is not very flexible—stretching it beyond its capacity can result in inflammation, ruptures, or tears. Although Achilles tendonitis is a chronic injury, its symptoms can come on suddenly or appear if a bout of acute tendonitis fails to heal properly. If you suspect that you may have developed this injury, don't try to push through the pain; instead stop and rest immediately.

Causes

- Lack of flexibility in the calf muscles
- Excessive training or overuse

Symptoms

- Pain in the back of the ankle and just above the heel
- Pain that increases during running
- Pain that eases as you warm up and stretch the tendon
- Pinpoint tenderness or soreness that increases when palpated
- Small lumps and bumps over the area of the tendon

Treatment

- Reducing your running routine
- Avoiding speed training and hill running
- Pre-run stretching exercises
- Post-run cold packs

BLISTERS

These fluid-filled sacks on the surface of the skin, caused by friction between skin and shoes/socks, can ruin anyone's run. Not only are blisters painful, they can also alter your gait, which may lead to more serious injuries of the leg and hip. To reduce friction, wear well-fitted shoes and seamless, moisture-wicking socks. Try spreading petroleum jelly on blister-prone areas, too.

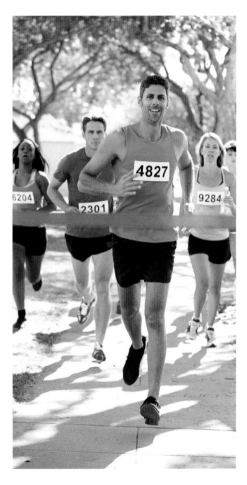

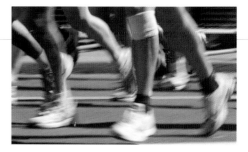

Muscle strain

Some of the most common injuries runners suffer are muscle strains, also called muscle pulls. These are small tears in a muscle, caused by stretching the fibers beyond capacity. The hamstrings, quadriceps, calf muscles, and groin muscles are the most frequent sites of strains. A popping sensation in the affected area is a typical sign that you have strained a muscle.

Causes
• Overstretching a muscle
• Excessive training or overuse
• Fatigue
• Falling

Symptoms
• A sudden, sharp pain in the affected area
• Muscle stiffness, soreness and tightness
• Swelling or bruising (moderate and severe strains)

Treatment
• Rest
• Cold packs
• Compression
• Elevation of affected area

Lower-back pain

Running often places stress on the lower back, and the repetitive motion may aggravate existing lumbar problems or even bring on persistent or intermittent lower-back pain.

Causes
• Tight or weak lower-back muscles

Symptoms
• Pain and stiffness in the lumbar area
  • Pain or a tingling sensation running from the lower back through the leg

Treatment
  • Warming up before running
• Stretching exercises
• Strengthening exercises
• Wearing properly fitted running-specific shoes
• Running on forgiving surfaces
• Cold packs

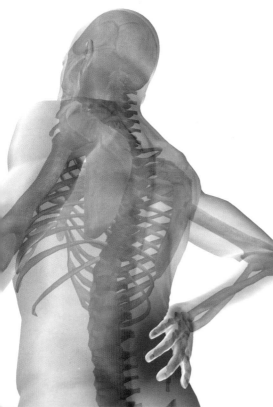

MUSCLE ACTIVATION & THE GAIT CYCLE

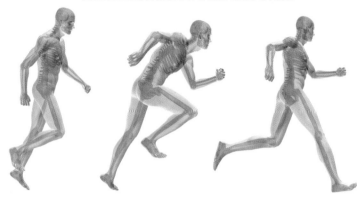

Running may be a natural human activity, but to derive the most benefit from running, proper form is essential. The first step is to understand the gait cycle, or the rhythmic alternating movements of the legs and feet that result in the forward movement of the body—in other words, how you run. A gait cycle begins when one foot makes contact with the ground and ends when that same foot makes contact with the ground again. It consists of two phases: the stance (or support) phase and the swing (or unsupported) phase. A running gait consists of the following:

Stance phase. Begins when the heel of the forward leg makes contact with the ground and ends when the toe of the same leg leaves the ground. This phase has three subphases:
- *Heel strike.* The heel of the forward foot touches the ground.
- *Midstance.* The foot is flat on the ground, and the weight of the body is directly over the supporting limb. In midstance, as your other foot is in swing phase, all your body weight is borne by a single leg, which means that the lower leg is particularly susceptible to injury.
- *Toe-off.* Only the big toe of the forward foot is in contact with the ground. During toe-off, your foot should be supinated (rotated outward), allowing the bones of the midfoot to brace against each other, which forms a rigid structure that propels the body weight forward. Improper running shoes or an abnormally pronating foot can prevent the correct functioning of the foot in

this phase, increasing the risk of injury. The quadriceps and rectus femoris work as knee extensors, while the rectus femoris also contributes to hip flexion. These muscles engage in anticipation of and during the stance phase to support the body. The rectus femoris also activates in mid-swing phase to flex the hip.

Swing phase. Begins when the foot is no longer in contact with the ground. The leg is free to move. This phase has two subphases:
- *Acceleration.* The swinging limb catches up to and passes the torso.
- *Deceleration.* Forward movement of the limb is slowed down to position the foot for heel strike.

Most muscles work in pairs, with an antagonist muscle working in opposition to an agonist. The major antagonist muscles to the quadriceps are the gluteal muscles, which extend the hip, and the hamstrings, which extend the hip and flex the knee. The hamstring muscles activate in mid-swing phase to help decelerate the lower leg. In late swing phase and in the first half of the stance phase, both groups engage to begin extending the hip.

Lower-leg muscles acting on the ankle are the tibialis anterior, gastrocnemius, and soleus. The gastrocnemius and soleus are active in the last part of swing phase to prepare for foot strike and remain active through the stance phase until just before toe-off, so as to propel the body forward.

FULL-BODY ANATOMY

FRONT

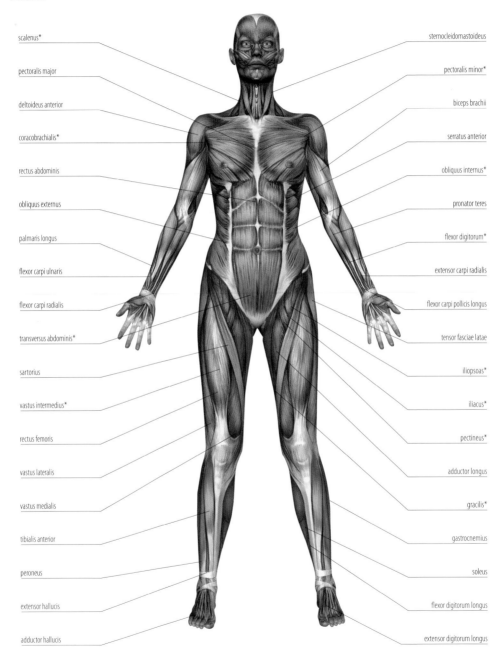

scalenus*

pectoralis major

deltoideus anterior

coracobrachialis*

rectus abdominis

obliquus externus

palmaris longus

flexor carpi ulnaris

flexor carpi radialis

transversus abdominis*

sartorius

vastus intermedius*

rectus femoris

vastus lateralis

vastus medialis

tibialis anterior

peroneus

extensor hallucis

adductor hallucis

sternocleidomastoideus

pectoralis minor*

biceps brachii

serratus anterior

obliquus internus*

pronator teres

flexor digitorum*

extensor carpi radialis

flexor carpi pollicis longus

tensor fasciae latae

iliopsoas*

iliacus*

pectineus*

adductor longus

gracilis*

gastrocnemius

soleus

flexor digitorum longus

extensor digitorum longus

ANNOTATION KEY

* indicates deep muscles

BACK

semispinalis*

trapezius

deltoideus medialis

infraspinatus*

deltoideus posterior

teres minor

subscapularis*

triceps brachii

rhomboideus*

anconeus

multifidus spinae*

gemellus superior*

quadratus femoris*

obturator internus*

obturator externus

vastus lateralis

gemellus inferior*

adductor magnus

plantaris

gastrocnemius

soleus

flexor digitorum longus

splenius*

levator scapulae*

supraspinatus*

teres major

erector spinae*

brachialis

latissimus dorsi

brachioradialis

extensor digitorum

quadratus lumborum*

gluteus minimus*

gluteus medius*

piriformis*

tractus iliotibialis

gluteus maximus

semitendinosus

biceps femoris

semimembranosus

tibialis posterior*

flexor hallucis*

trochlea tali

adductor digiti minimi

ANNOTATION KEY

* indicates deep muscles

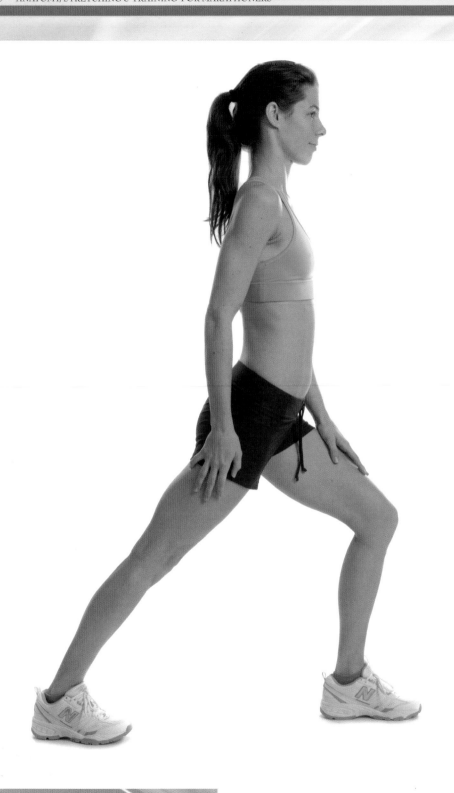

RUNNERS' STRETCHES

As with any kind of exercise, before setting off on a run, it is important to warm up and stretch your muscles. Stretching exercises lengthen the muscle fibers, increasing their functionality. With regular pre-run and post-run stretching, you will see not only greater flexibility but also improved posture, balance, and range of motion. The following pages feature stretches that focus on the primary running muscles—the quadriceps, hamstrings, glutes, calves, ankles, and hip flexors, as well as secondary areas such as the lumbar spine.

For optimum results, do a fast 5-to-10-minute cardiovascular warm-up, and then perform a series of these stretches before a run. After a run, a few of these stretches will form a perfect cool-down regimen.

STANDING QUADS STRETCH

BEGINNER

The quadriceps femoris group are the long muscles that sit on the front aspect of your thigh. It is essential for you to stretch this major group of primary running muscles in order to achieve full length and flexibility in your legs. During this stretch, be sure to stand tall, without leaning or rocking, to improve your balance as well.

ANNOTATION KEY

Black text indicates strengthening muscles
Gray text indicates stretching muscles
Italic text indicates tendons and ligaments
- - - - indicates deep muscles

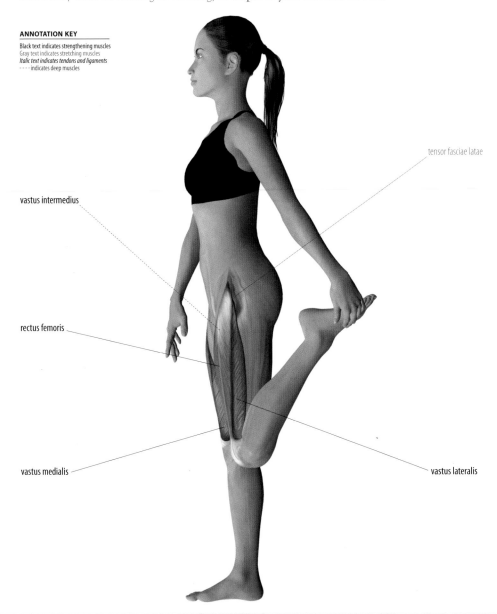

tensor fasciae latae

vastus intermedius

rectus femoris

vastus medialis

vastus lateralis

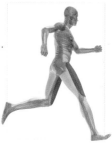

HOW TO DO IT

1 Stand with your feet together. Bend your left leg behind you, and grasp your foot with your left hand. Pull your heel toward your buttocks until you feel a stretch in the front of your thigh. Keep both knees together and aligned.

2 Hold for 15 seconds. Repeat sequence three times on each leg.

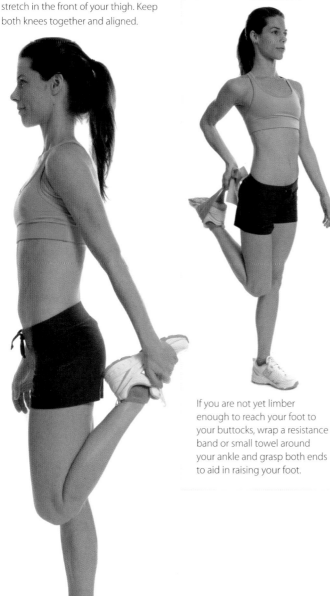

If you are not yet limber enough to reach your foot to your buttocks, wrap a resistance band or small towel around your ankle and grasp both ends to aid in raising your foot.

PRIMARY TARGETS
- rectus femoris
- vastus lateralis
- vastus medialis
- vastus intermedius

BENEFITS
- Helps to keep thigh muscles flexible

CAUTIONS
- Knee issues

PERFECT YOUR FORM
- Both knees should remain pressed together.
- With your arm opposite the bent leg, lean against a wall or other stable object to aid your balance.
- Avoid leaning forward with your chest.
- Avoid bringing your foot closer to your buttocks than you can reach with a comfortable, pain-free stretch—this can compress the knee joint.

SPRINTER'S STRETCH

BEGINNER

RUNNING PLACES STRAIN on both your Achilles tendon (the large tendon running from your heel to your calf) and the soleus (the muscle running between the two heads of the large gastrocnemius muscle of your calf). The Sprinter's Stretch works on both, helping you to avoid common running injuries, such as Achilles tendonitis.

ANNOTATION KEY
Black text indicates strengthening muscles
Gray text indicates stretching muscles
Italic text indicates tendons and ligaments
---- indicates deep muscles

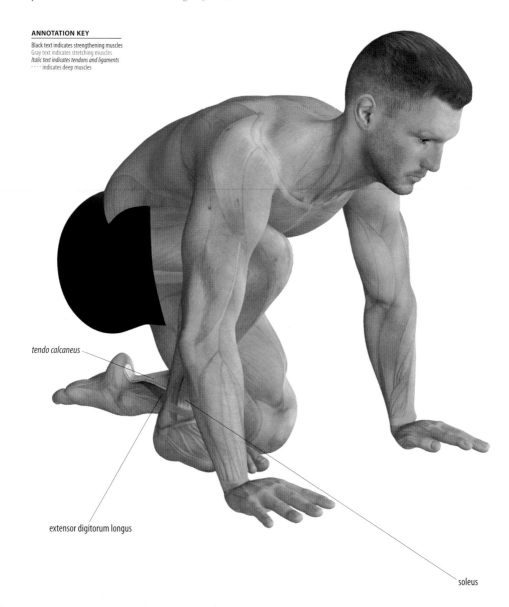

tendo calcaneus

extensor digitorum longus

soleus

HOW TO DO IT

1 Kneel with your left knee bent, your toe pointed and extended behind you on the floor. Bend your right leg so that your right foot is flat on the floor, next to your left knee.

2 Place your palms on the floor just beyond shoulder-width apart, slightly in front of your body.

3 Sit back on your right heel as you lean slightly forward.

4 Release the stretch, switch legs, and repeat on the other side.

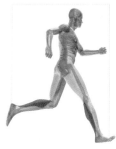

PRIMARY TARGETS

- tendo calcaneus
- extensor digitorum longus
- soleus

BENEFITS

- Strengthens and stretches the Achilles tendon
- Stretches calf muscles

CAUTIONS

- Knee issues

PERFECT YOUR FORM

- Keep the sole of your front foot and the upper arch of your back foot on the floor.
- Lean your chest farther forward over your raised upper leg to increase the intensity of the stretch.
- Avoid allowing your foot to roll inwards.

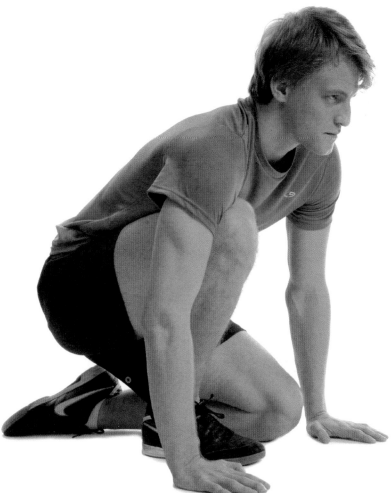

FORWARD LUNGE

BEGINNER

THE FORWARD LUNGE is an excellent stretching exercise that targets your glutes and your quadriceps, along with your hamstrings, soleus, and gastrocnemius muscles. All these groups are primary running muscles, and keeping them in top condition will allow you to run farther for longer stretches of time.

ANNOTATION KEY
Black text indicates strengthening muscles
Gray text indicates stretching muscles
Italic text indicates tendons and ligaments
- - - - indicates deep muscles

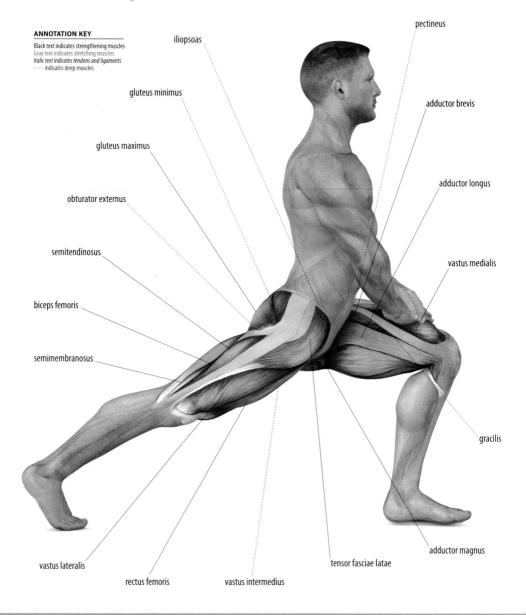

pectineus

iliopsoas

gluteus minimus

adductor brevis

gluteus maximus

obturator externus

adductor longus

semitendinosus

vastus medialis

biceps femoris

semimembranosus

gracilis

vastus lateralis

rectus femoris

vastus intermedius

tensor fasciae latae

adductor magnus

HOW TO DO IT

1 Stand with your legs and feet parallel and shoulder-width apart, and your knees bent very slightly. Tuck your pelvis slightly forward, lift your chest, and press your shoulders downward and back.

2 Bend your left knee, and step your right leg back behind your body, extending it straight.

3 Place your palms on your knee, and hold for 15 seconds.

4 Release the stretch, switch legs, and repeat on the other side.

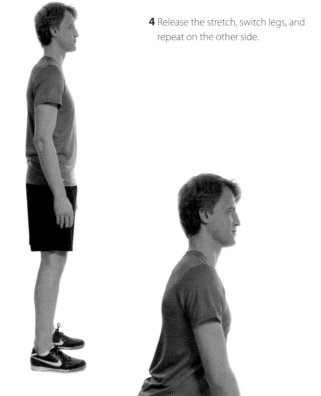

PRIMARY TARGETS

• rectus femoris
• vastus lateralis
• vastus intermedius
• vastus medialis
• biceps femoris
• semitendinosus
• semimembranosus
• gluteus maximus
• adductor longus
• adductor magnus
• adductor brevis
• iliopsoas
• gracilis
• pectineus
• tensor fasciae latae
• obturator externus
• gluteus minimus

BENEFITS

• Stretches hip flexors
• Strengthens hamstrings, thighs, and glutes

CAUTIONS

• Severe hip or knee degeneration

PERFECT YOUR FORM

• Keep your back leg extended in line with your hips to form one long straight line.
• Keep your knee directly above your ankle.
• Avoid dropping your back extended leg to the floor.
• Avoid hunching your shoulders.

STRAIGHT-LEG LUNGE

BEGINNER

It is quite common for marathon and distance runners to develop "quad dominance," which means that their quadriceps overpower the action of their hamstrings muscles during a running stride, putting them at risk for hamstrings injuries. The Straight-Leg Lunge focuses its attention on your hamstrings, both stretching and strengthening them.

ANNOTATION KEY
Black text indicates strengthening muscles
Gray text indicates stretching muscles
Italic text indicates tendons and ligaments
- - - - indicates deep muscles

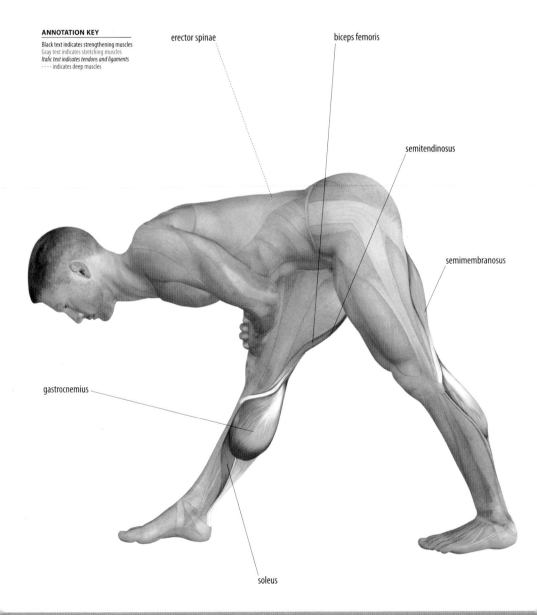

erector spinae

biceps femoris

semitendinosus

semimembranosus

gastrocnemius

soleus

HOW TO DO IT

1 Stand with your legs and feet parallel and shoulder-width apart. Bend your knees very slightly and tuck your pelvis slightly forward, lift your chest, and press your shoulders downward and back.

2 Leading with your right foot, take one step forward.

3 Keeping your legs straight, lean your torso forward as far as possible over your right leg. Allow the weight of your upper body to intensify the stretch.

4 Return to standing, and repeat on the other side.

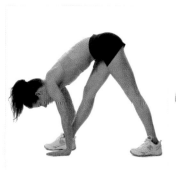

Challenge yourself with a deeper stretch by placing your hands flat on the floor on either side of your front foot.

PRIMARY TARGETS
• biceps femoris
• semitendinosus
• semimembranosus
• erector spinae
• gastrocnemius
• soleus

BENEFITS
• Stretches hamstrings, calves, and lower back

CAUTIONS
• Lower-back pain

PERFECT YOUR FORM
• Flex your front foot by lifting the ball of your foot off the floor to maximize the intensity of the stretch.
• Keep the heel of your back leg on the floor throughout the stretch.
• Let go of any unnecessary tension in the upper body— relax and breathe in and out naturally.

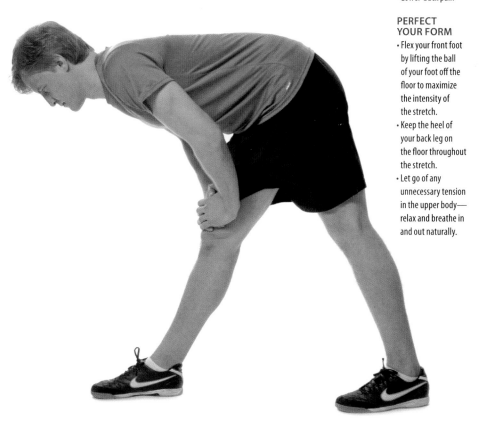

WIDE-LEGGED FORWARD BEND

BEGINNER

THE WIDE-LEGGED FORWARD BEND stretches your entire body, with particular focus on your hamstrings and spine. Known also as Wide-Angle Standing Forward Bend and Standing Straddle Forward Bend, this exercise has its origins in yoga, which is famous for keeping its practitioners limber and strong.

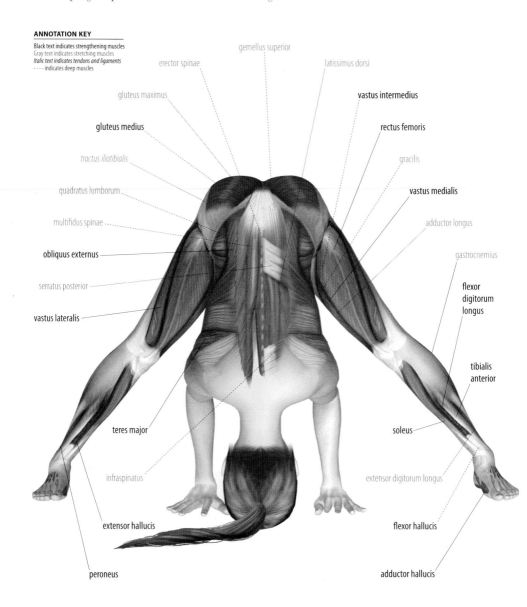

ANNOTATION KEY

Black text indicates strengthening muscles
Gray text indicates stretching muscles
Italic text indicates tendons and ligaments
---- indicates deep muscles

gemellus superior

erector spinae

latissimus dorsi

gluteus maximus

vastus intermedius

gluteus medius

rectus femoris

tractus iliotibialis

gracilis

quadratus lumborum

vastus medialis

multifidus spinae

adductor longus

obliquus externus

gastrocnemius

serratus posterior

flexor digitorum longus

vastus lateralis

tibialis anterior

teres major

soleus

infraspinatus

extensor digitorum longus

extensor hallucis

flexor hallucis

peroneus

adductor hallucis

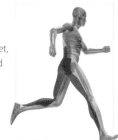

HOW TO DO IT

1 Stand with your legs and feet parallel and generously outside of shoulder width. Bend your knees very slightly and tuck your pelvis slightly forward, lift your chest, and press your shoulders downward and back.

2 Exhale, and bend forward from your hips, keeping your back flat. Draw your sternum forward as you lower your torso, gazing straight ahead. With your elbows straight, place your fingertips or palms on the floor.

3 With another exhalation, place your hands on the floor in between your feet, and lower your torso into a full forward bend. Lengthen your spine by pulling your sit bones up toward the ceiling and drawing your head to the floor. If possible, bend your elbows and place your forehead on the floor.

4 Hold for 30 seconds to 1 minute. To return to your starting position, straighten your elbows and raise your torso while keeping your back flat.

PRIMARY TARGETS
- biceps femoris
- semitendinosus
- semimembranosus
- gluteus maximus
- gluteus medius
- gluteus minimus
- rectus abdominis
- transversus abdominis
- obliquus externus
- obliquus internus
- erector spinae
- gastrocnemius
- soleus

BENEFITS
- Stretches and strengthens hamstrings, groins, and spine

CAUTIONS
- Lower-back issues

PERFECT YOUR FORM
- Contract your leg muscles, and keep your feet firmly grounded throughout the stretch.
- Keep your chest elevated.
- Avoid tensing your shoulders.

If your back or hamstrings are tight, try this easier version: Follow step 1, and then exhale, bending forward until your torso is nearly parallel to the floor. Place your hands on the floor in line with your shoulders, making sure that your lower back is straight. Hold for 15 to 30 seconds.

Another easy modification calls for you to widen your stance or place a block, book, or other solid object on the floor for support.

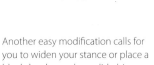

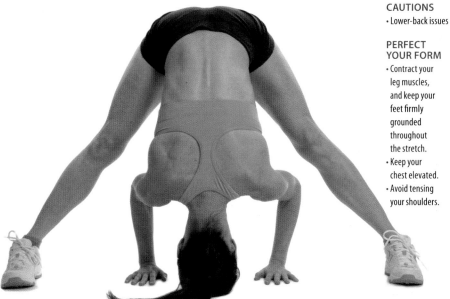

BILATERAL SEATED FORWARD BEND

BEGINNER

YOUR HAMSTRINGS BEND YOUR KNEES, extend your hips, and rotate your thighs. Weak or tight hamstrings are a runner's enemy, disrupting the muscular balance of your entire body. To prepare for a run, use stretches such as the Bilateral Seated Forward Bend to keep your hamstrings—along with your back, calf, and groin muscles—limber.

ANNOTATION KEY

Black text indicates strengthening muscles
Gray text indicates stretching muscles
Italic text indicates tendons and ligaments
- - - - indicates deep muscles

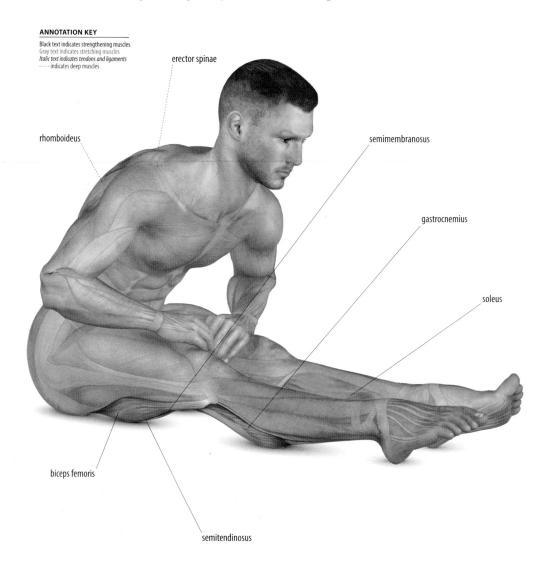

erector spinae

rhomboideus

semimembranosus

gastrocnemius

soleus

biceps femoris

semitendinosus

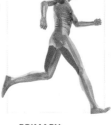

HOW TO DO IT

1 Sit on the floor, sitting up as straight as possible with your back flattened and your legs extended in front of you in parallel position. Your feet should be relaxed and flexed slightly.

2 Lean forward, lowering your abdominals over your thighs, forearms resting above your kneecaps as you stretch.

3 Slowly roll up, and repeat if desired.

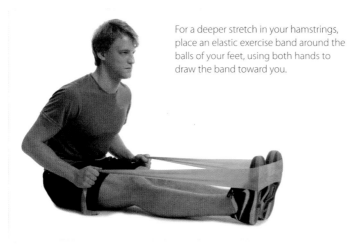

For a deeper stretch in your hamstrings, place an elastic exercise band around the balls of your feet, using both hands to draw the band toward you.

PRIMARY TARGETS
- biceps femoris
- semitendinosus
- semimembranosus
- multifidus spinae
- erector spinae
- gastrocnemius
- soleus
- rhomboideus

BENEFITS
- Stretches hamstrings, groin, and spine

CAUTIONS
- Headache

PERFECT YOUR FORM
- Bend at the hips and keep your spine straight as you stretch.
- Extend your torso as far forward over your legs as possible.
- Don't hold your breath.
- Don't tense your jaw or clench your teeth while performing any stretch: relaxing your mouth will help you breathe evenly.

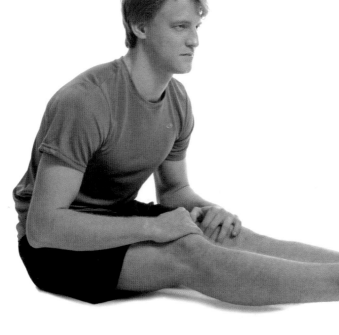

UNILATERAL SEATED FORWARD BEND

BEGINNER

As its name implies, in the Unilateral Seated Forward Bend, you extend only one leg forward during the stretch. As well as focusing on your hamstrings, the Unilateral Seated Forward Bend works as a spinal twist, especially in the advanced version. If you are just beginning a running regimen, you can hook a strap around your extended foot and hold an end in each hand as you bend forward.

ANNOTATION KEY

Black text indicates strengthening muscles
Gray text indicates stretching muscles
Italic text indicates tendons and ligaments
- - - - indicates deep muscles

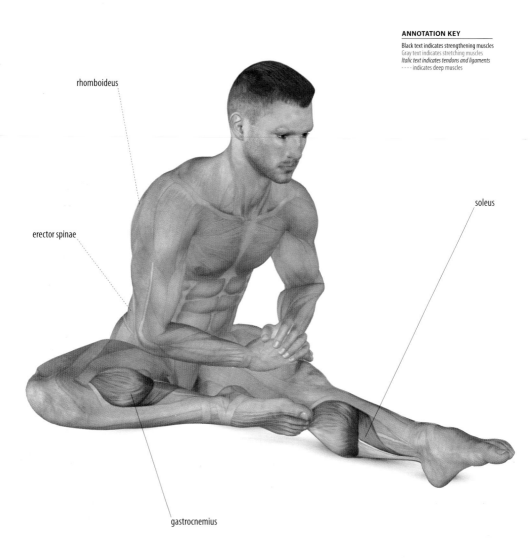

rhomboideus

soleus

erector spinae

gastrocnemius

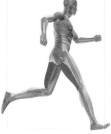

HOW TO DO IT

1 Sit on the floor, back straight and with your legs extended in front of you in parallel position.

2 Bend your right leg outward, with the bottom of your right foot resting at your left inner thigh just above the kneecap. Rest your hands on your knee.

3 Bend from your waist, and lean forward over your left leg. Place your forearms above your left kneecap.

4 Hold for 10 to 30 seconds.

5 Switch legs, and repeat the stretch on the other side.

To challenge yourself with a deeper forward bend, follow steps 1 through 3, then exhale and stretch your sternum forward as you fold your torso over your left leg. Grasp the inside of your left foot with your right hand. Use your left hand to guide your torso to the left.

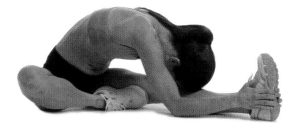

PRIMARY TARGETS
• biceps femoris
• semitendinosus
• semimembranosus
• multifidus spinae
• erector spinae
• gastrocnemius
• soleus
• rhomboideus

BENEFITS
• Stretches hamstrings, groin, and spine

CAUTIONS
• Knee injury
• Lower-back injury

PERFECT YOUR FORM
• Drop your head to benefit your rhomboids and for a more intense overall stretch.
• Avoid allowing the foot of your bent leg to shift beneath your straight leg.
• Avoid straining your back—if yours is tight, try performing this stretch with a support, such as a sofa, behind you. Be sure to position your lower back as close to the support as possible.

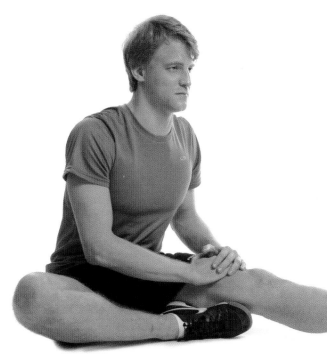

KNEE-TO-CHEST HUG

BEGINNER

The Knee-to-Chest Hug stretches and strengthens your lower-back muscles and stretches your glutes. Perform it after a run to ease any strain placed on your back, with your shoulders relaxed and hips firmly grounded. And remember: stretch only until you feel very mild discomfort—never to the point of pain.

ANNOTATION KEY

Black text indicates strengthening muscles
Gray text indicates stretching muscles
Italic text indicates tendons and ligaments
- - - - indicates deep muscles

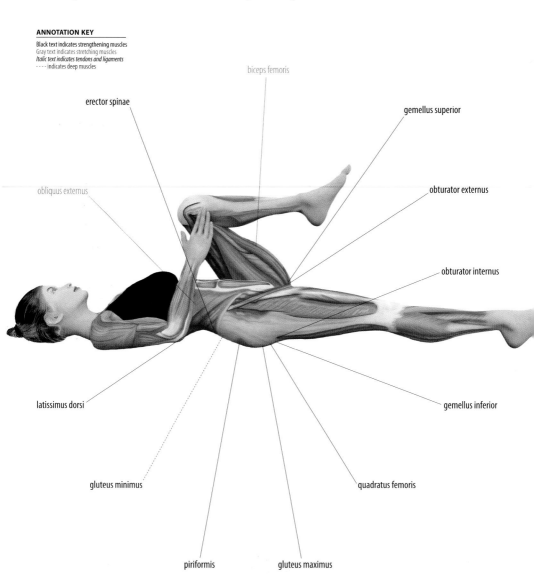

biceps femoris

erector spinae

gemellus superior

obliquus externus

obturator externus

obturator internus

latissimus dorsi

gemellus inferior

gluteus minimus

quadratus femoris

piriformis

gluteus maximus

HOW TO DO IT

1 Lie supine on a mat with your legs together and arms outstretched.

2 Bend your right knee, and bring your foot to your body's midline while clasping your hands together to hold your knee. Hold the stretch for 15 seconds.

3 Return to the starting position.

4 Again, clasping your hands together to hold your knee, bend your right knee, but this time rotate the right leg to the left, bringing the side of your leg against your chest.

5 Hold the stretch for 15 seconds, and then return to the starting position. Repeat the entire sequence with the left leg bent.

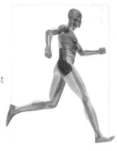

PRIMARY TARGETS
- erector spinae
- latissimus dorsi
- gluteus maximus
- gluteus minimus
- piriformis
- gemellus superior
- gemellus inferior
- obturator externus
- obturator internus
- quadratus femoris

BENEFITS
- Stretches lower back, hip extensors, and hip rotators

CAUTIONS
- Advanced degenerative joint disease

PERFECT YOUR FORM
- Keep your spine in neutral position.
- Lift your buttocks off the floor.

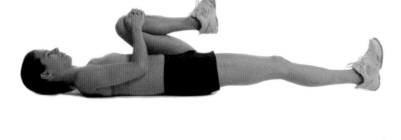

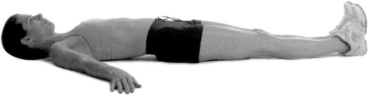

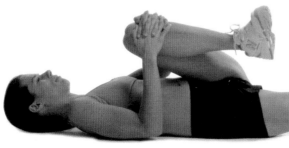

SUPINE FIGURE 4

BEGINNER

THE PIRIFORMIS IS A SMALL pear-shaped muscle, lying deep behind the gluteals, which rotates your hips. If your piriformis muscle becomes too tight, it can impinge on your sciatic nerve, resulting in pain radiating from your buttocks, down your thigh, and up into your spine. Supine Figure 4 targets this important muscle, so lie flat on a mat, distributing your weight evenly to obtain an effective, controlled stretch.

ANNOTATION KEY

Black text indicates strengthening muscles
Gray text indicates stretching muscles
Italic text indicates tendons and ligaments
----indicates deep muscles

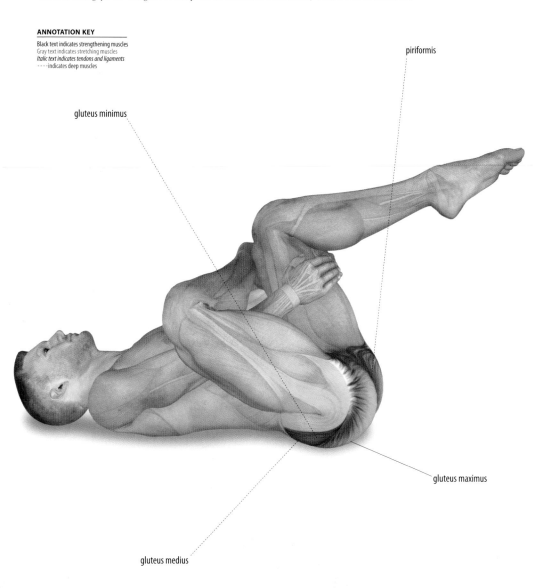

piriformis

gluteus minimus

gluteus maximus

gluteus medius

HOW TO DO IT

1 Lie on your back with your legs extended and toes pointed.

2 Bend your right knee and turn your leg out so that your right ankle rests on your left thigh just above the knee, creating a the shape of a figure 4

3 Bend your left leg, drawing both legs (still in the figure 4 position) in toward

your chest as you grasp the back of your left thigh.

4 Push your right elbow against your right inner thigh, slightly turning out your right leg to increase the intensity of the stretch.

6 Return to the starting position, switch legs, and repeat.

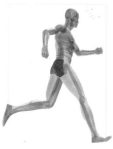

PRIMARY TARGETS
• gluteus maximus
• gluteus medius
• gluteus minimus
• piriformis

BENEFITS
• Stretches glutes and lower back

CAUTIONS
• Knee issues
• Severe lower-back pain

PERFECT YOUR FORM
• Keep your head and shoulder blades on the floor.
• Relax your hips so that you can go deeper into the stretch.
• Perform the stretch slowly.

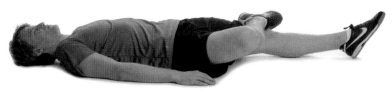

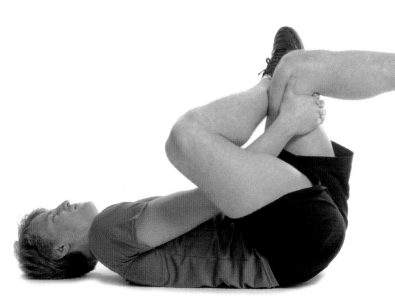

SIDE-LYING KNEE BEND

BEGINNER

LIKE THE STANDING QUADS STRETCH, the Side-Lying Knee Bend targets the quadriceps muscles of the front of your thigh—the rectus femoris, vastus intermedius, vastus lateralis, and vastus medialis. Running strengthens these muscles, but can also tighten them, so be sure to stretch them regularly to keep them limber and flexible.

ANNOTATION KEY
Black text indicates strengthening muscles
Gray text indicates stretching muscles
Italic text indicates tendons and ligaments
- - - -indicates deep muscles

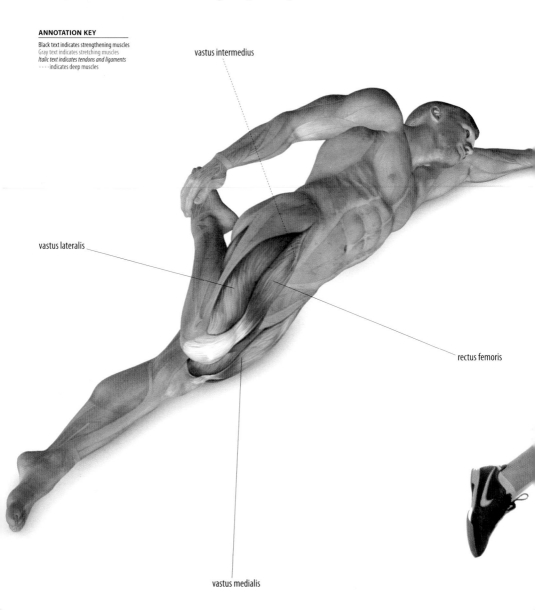

vastus intermedius

vastus lateralis

rectus femoris

vastus medialis

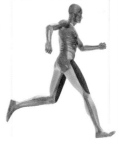

HOW TO DO IT

1 Lie on your left side, with your legs extended together in line with your body. Extend your left arm, and rest your head on your upper arm.

2 Bend your right knee and grasp your ankle with your right hand.

3 Pull your ankle in toward your buttocks as you stretch.

4 Return to the starting position, and repeat on the other side.

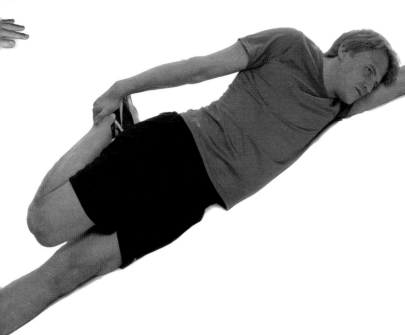

PRIMARY TARGETS
- rectus femoris
- vastus lateralis
- vastus intermedius
- vastus medialis

BENEFITS
- Helps to keep thigh muscles flexible

CAUTIONS
- Knee issues

PERFECT YOUR FORM
- Keep your knees together, one on top of the other.
- Tuck your pelvis slightly forward, and lift your chest to engage and stretch your core.
- Keep your foot pointed and parallel with your leg.
- Avoid leaning back onto your glutes.
- Place a towel under your bottom hip if it feels uncomfortable to rest directly on the floor.

SIDE-LYING RIB STRETCH

BEGINNER

EXERCISES SUCH AS THE SIDE-LYING RIB STRETCH are runners' essentials because they lengthen the muscles between the ribs and pelvis and open the sides of the rib cage, which improves rib-cage mobility and increases lung expansion. This makes breathing—a critical component of aerobic activities such as marathon running—easier.

ANNOTATION KEY

Black text indicates strengthening muscles
Gray text indicates stretching muscles
Italic text indicates tendons and ligaments
- - - - indicates deep muscles

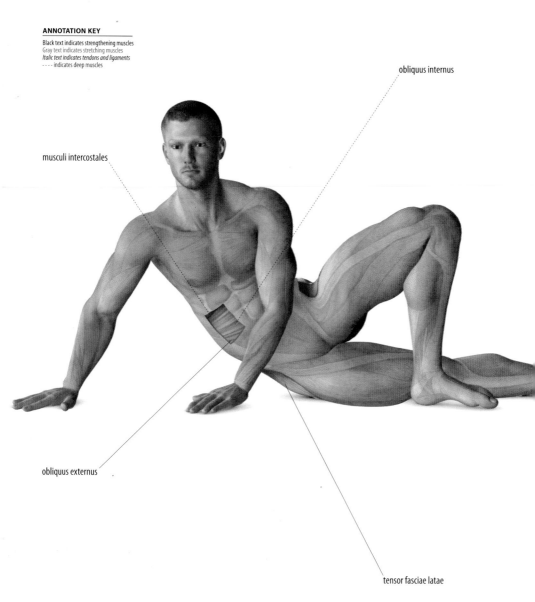

obliquus internus

musculi intercostales

obliquus externus

tensor fasciae latae

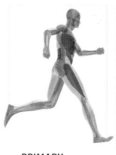

HOW TO DO IT

1 Lie on your right side with your legs together and extended. Place both palms on the floor, your right arm supporting you and your left arm positioned in front of your body. Your upper body should be slightly lifted.

2 Bend your left leg and rest the foot just in front of your right thigh, knee pointing up toward the ceiling.

3 Keeping your legs in place, press down with your hands and straighten both your arms as you raise your body upward, feeling a stretch around your right side and rib cage.

4 Release, switch sides, and repeat.

PRIMARY TARGETS

- obliquus externus
- obliquus internus
- tensor fasciae latae
- multifidus spinae
- erector spinae

BENEFITS

- Strengthens lower back, obliques, and outer thighs

CAUTIONS

- Severe lower-back pain

PERFECT YOUR FORM

- Shift your weight forward on your supporting hip.
- Place a towel under your bottom hip if you are uncomfortable resting directly on the floor.
- Don't tighten your jaw muscles, which can cause tension in your neck.

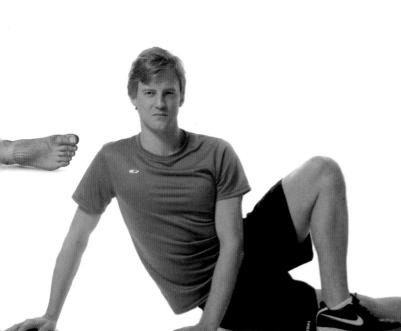

HEEL-DROP/TOE-UP STRETCH

BEGINNER

THE HEEL-DROP/TOE-UP STRETCH will work your gastrocnemius, soleus, and Achilles tendon. Stretching and strengthening the muscles and tendons of your calves should be a consistent part of your running exercise regimen. When properly toned, your calf muscles help keep you balanced while running, while also contributing to your ankle strength.

ANNOTATION KEY

Black text indicates strengthening muscles
Gray text indicates stretching muscles
Italic text indicates tendons and ligaments
- - - - indicates deep muscles

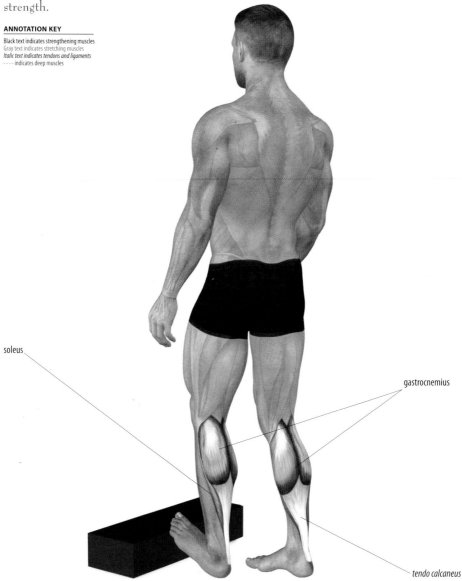

soleus

gastrocnemius

tendo calcaneus

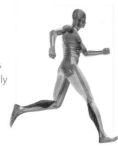

HOW TO DO IT

1 Stand on an aerobic step, a riser, or a stair with your legs and feet parallel and shoulder-width apart. Bend your knees very slightly and tuck your pelvis slightly forward, lift your chest, and press your shoulders downward and back.

2 Position your left foot slightly in front of your right, and place the ball of your right foot on the edge of the step.

3 Drop your right heel down while controlling the amount of weight on the right leg to increase or decrease the intensity of the stretch in the right calf.

4 Release, switch feet, and repeat on the other side.

5 Step down from the riser, and stand with your legs and feet parallel and shoulder-width apart. Bend your knees very slightly and tuck your pelvis slightly forward, lift your chest, and press your shoulders downward and back.

6 Position the ball of your left foot on the step.

7 With your knees straight, bring your hips forward.

8 Release, switch feet, and repeat on the other side.

PRIMARY TARGETS
• gastrocnemius
• soleus
• tendo calcaneus

BENEFITS
• Stretches calf muscles and Achilles tendon

CAUTIONS
• Strained calf muscle

PERFECT YOUR FORM
• Use a wall or other stable object to balance yourself if necessary.
• Engage your entire calf muscle by gently and slowly rolling from your big toe to your small toe and back again, shifting your body weight over your toes as you go.
• Avoid bouncing to achieve a greater stretch—all of your movements should be performed slowly and carefully.

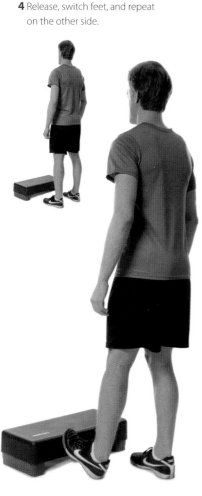

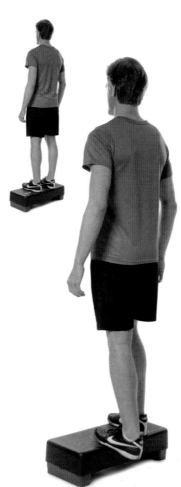

CALF STRETCH

BEGINNER

WHETHER DEDICATED MARATHONERS or casual joggers, all runners rely on this stretch for full-leg flexibility. In its first part, with your forward leg straight, you will target your gastrocnemius, the large bifurcated muscle at the back of your calf. With a bend of the knee, your focus shifts to the soleus muscle. This stretch improves flexibility and can also improve running speed.

ANNOTATION KEY

Black text indicates strengthening muscles
Gray text indicates stretching muscles
Italic text indicates tendons and ligaments
- - - - indicates deep muscles

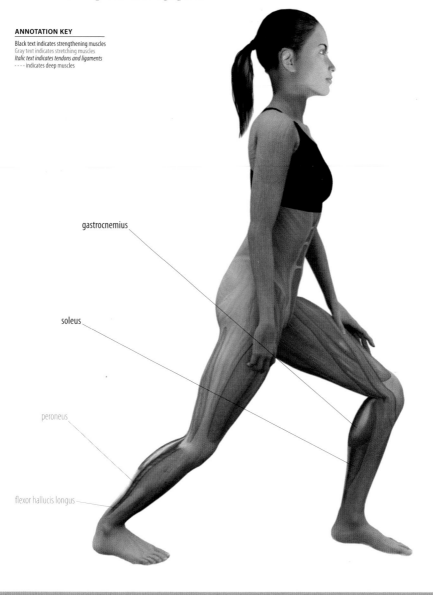

gastrocnemius

soleus

peroneus

flexor hallucis longus

HOW TO DO IT

1 Stand with your legs straight, one foot behind the other.

2 Bring your front leg forward and bend your front knee.

3 Keeping both heels on the floor, lean into your front leg until you feel the stretch in your back calf muscle. Hold for 15 seconds. Repeat sequence three times on each leg.

4 With your foot still forward and your front knee still bent, keep both heels on the floor, and lean into the stretch as you bend your back knee. Switch legs and repeat sequence three times.

5 Once you feel the stretch, hold the position for 15 seconds. Repeat stretch three times on each leg.

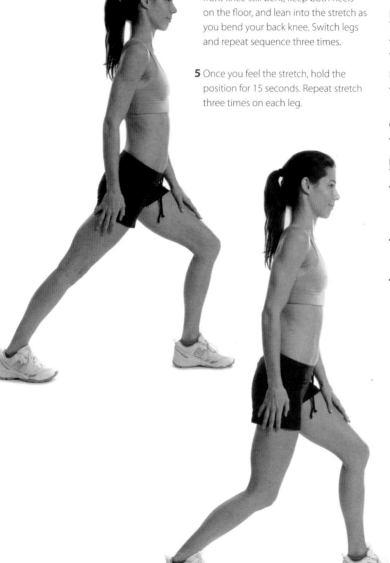

RUNNERS' STRETCHES

PRIMARY TARGETS
• soleus
• gastrocnemius

BENEFITS
• Stretches your calf muscles

CAUTIONS
• Strained calf muscle

PERFECT YOUR FORM
• Keep your chest upright and lifted as you lean into the stretch.
• Avoid bending your extended leg during step 3.
• Avoid lifting your heel off the floor.

ILIOTIBIAL BAND STRETCH

BEGINNER

THE ILIOTIBIAL BAND IS a thick band of connective tissue that crosses your hip joint and extends down to insert on your kneecap, tibia, and biceps femoris tendon. The iliotibial band stabilizes your knee and abducts your hip. Perform the Iliotibial Band Stretch as a pre-run stretch and before attempting any of the more demanding lower-body exercises included in this book.

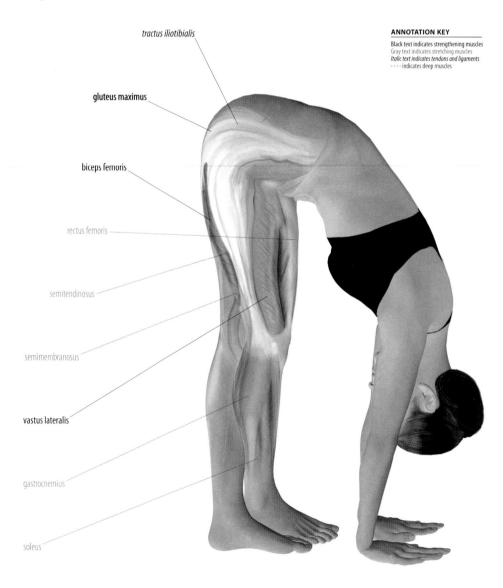

ANNOTATION KEY
Black text indicates strengthening muscles
Gray text indicates stretching muscles
Italic text indicates tendons and ligaments
---- indicates deep muscles

tractus iliotibialis

gluteus maximus

biceps femoris

rectus femoris

semitendinosus

semimembranosus

vastus lateralis

gastrocnemius

soleus

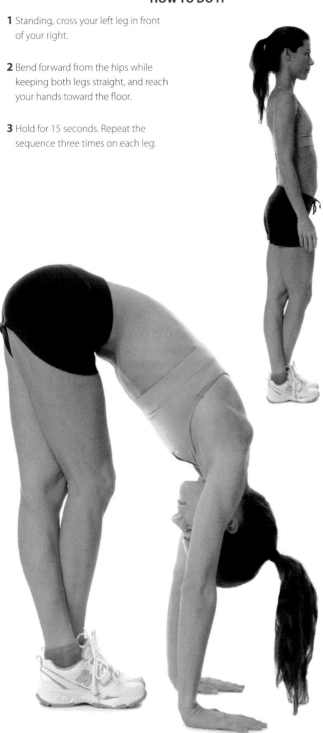

HOW TO DO IT

1 Standing, cross your left leg in front of your right.

2 Bend forward from the hips while keeping both legs straight, and reach your hands toward the floor.

3 Hold for 15 seconds. Repeat the sequence three times on each leg.

RUNNERS' STRETCHES

PRIMARY TARGETS
- tractus iliotibialis
- biceps femoris
- gluteus maximus
- vastus lateralis

BENEFITS
- Helps to stabilize knee joints
- Helps to keep hips flexible
- Stretches back, hamstrings, and calves

CAUTIONS
- Neck issues
- Lower-back pain

PERFECT YOUR FORM
- Keep both feet flat on the floor.
- Stretch with good alignment so that your back leg and your spine form a straight line.
- Avoid lifting your back heel off the floor.
- Avoid arching or round your back.

COBRA STRETCH

INTERMEDIATE

The Cobra Stretch takes its inspiration from the yoga pose that resembles the raised-hood stance of a cobra about to strike. When you properly execute this stretch, your body will take on the raised-hood position. It slowly stretches your entire spinal column and the muscles surrounding it, as well as stretches your glutes, chest, and abdominals.

ANNOTATION KEY

Black text indicates strengthening muscles
Gray text indicates stretching muscles
Italic text indicates tendons and ligaments
- - - -indicates deep muscles

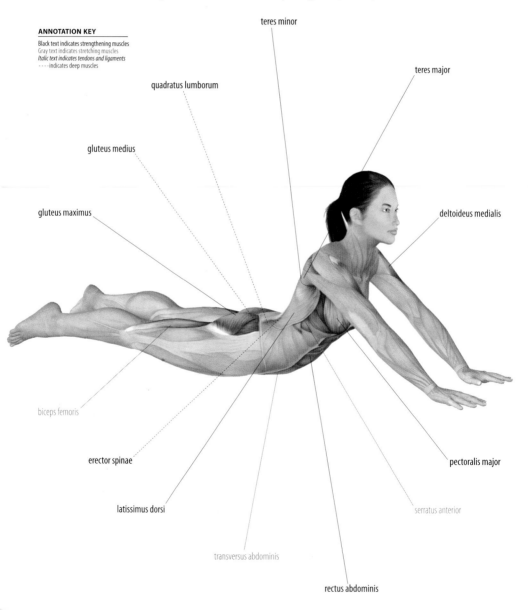

teres minor

teres major

quadratus lumborum

gluteus medius

gluteus maximus

deltoideus medialis

biceps femoris

erector spinae

pectoralis major

latissimus dorsi

serratus anterior

transversus abdominis

rectus abdominis

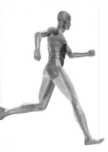

HOW TO DO IT

1 Lie prone on the floor. Bend your elbows, placing your hands flat on the floor beside your chest. Keep your elbows pulled in toward your body. Extend your legs, pressing your pubis, thighs, and tops of your feet into the floor.

2 Push down into the floor, and slowly lift through the top of your chest as you straighten your arms.

3 Pull your tailbone down toward your pubis as you push your shoulders down and back.

3 Elongate your neck and gaze forward.

5 Hold for 15 to 30 seconds, and exhale as you lower yourself to the floor.

PRIMARY TARGETS
- quadratus lumborum
- erector spinae
- latissimus dorsi
- gluteus maximus
- gluteus medius
- pectoralis major
- rectus abdominis
- deltoideus
- teres major
- teres minor

BENEFITS
- Strengthens spine and buttocks
- Stretches chest, abdominals, and shoulders

CAUTIONS
- Back injury

PERFECT YOUR FORM
- Lift out of your chest and back, rather than depending too much on your arms to create the arch in your back.
- Keep your shoulders and elbows pressed back to create more lift in your chest.
- Don't tense your buttocks, which adds pressure on your lower back.
- Avoid lifting your hips off the floor.

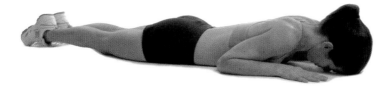

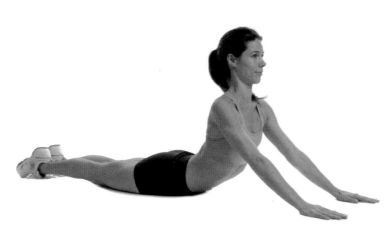

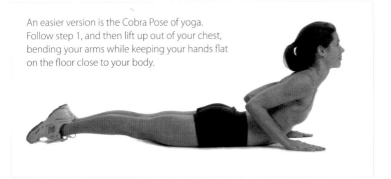

An easier version is the Cobra Pose of yoga. Follow step 1, and then lift up out of your chest, bending your arms while keeping your hands flat on the floor close to your body.

UNILATERAL LEG RAISE

INTERMEDIATE

THIS SIMPLE BUT EFFECTIVE STRETCH is important in preparing your lower back, hip extensors, and hip rotators for many of the more intensive exercises in this book. Take care not to overexert your hamstrings. Slow, deliberate stretching is best.

ANNOTATION KEY

Black text indicates strengthening muscles
Gray text indicates stretching muscles
Italic text indicates tendons and ligaments
- - - - indicates deep muscles

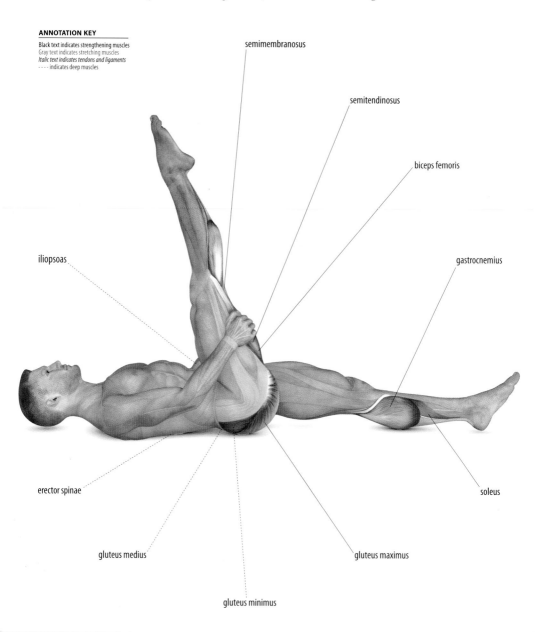

semimembranosus

semitendinosus

biceps femoris

iliopsoas

gastrocnemius

erector spinae

soleus

gluteus medius

gluteus maximus

gluteus minimus

RUNNERS' STRETCHES

HOW TO DO IT

1 Lie on your back with both legs extended and your spine in a imprinted position so that your lower back touches the floor.

2 With your hands placed on your hamstrings just below the knee, extend and straighten your left leg upward.

3 Point both feet, and hold this postion for 15 to 30 seconds.

4 Switch legs, and repeat the stretch on the other side.

PRIMARY TARGETS
- erector spinae
- gluteus maximus
- gluteus medius
- gluteus minimus
- biceps femoris
- semitendinosus
- semimembranosus
- iliopsoas
- gastrocnemius
- soleus

BENEFITS
- Stretches lower back, hip extensors, and hip rotators

CAUTIONS
- Advanced degenerative joint disease

PERFECT YOUR FORM
- Slightly tuck your pelvis to help keep your spine grounded and your lower back on the floor.
- Avoid lifting your head or upper back.
- Avoid holding your breath.

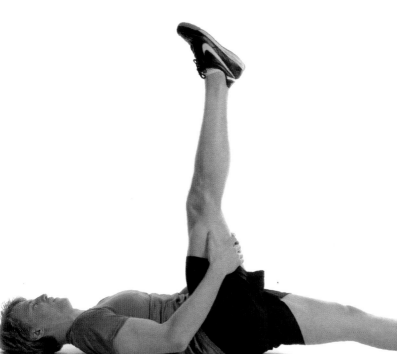

SPINAL ROTATION STRETCH

INTERMEDIATE

A LONG RUN CAN PLACE strain on your lower back, often leading to pain and tightness. A tight lower back also affects the muscles in your hips and thighs. The Spinal Rotation Stretch opens up your back and increases its flexibility. If you cannot reach your knees to the floor, try to get them as close as possible, making sure to keep your shoulders on the floor throughout the entire stretch.

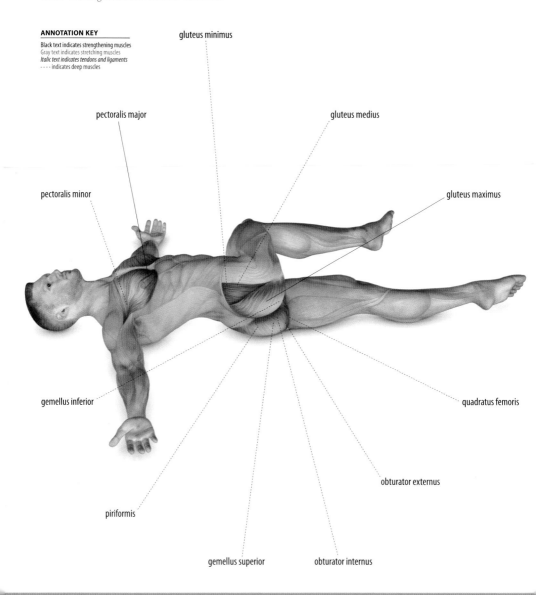

ANNOTATION KEY

Black text indicates strengthening muscles
Gray text indicates stretching muscles
Italic text indicates tendons and ligaments
- - - - indicates deep muscles

gluteus minimus

pectoralis major

gluteus medius

pectoralis minor

gluteus maximus

gemellus inferior

quadratus femoris

obturator externus

piriformis

gemellus superior

obturator internus

HOW TO DO IT

1 Lie on your back, with both legs elongated and parallel and your arms extended away from your torso, palms facing up.

2 Bend your right leg, placing the sole of your foot on the floor.

3 Carefully lift your buttocks off the floor, tilting your torso slightly to your left, and cross your right leg over to your left side, with your knee bent at a right angle.

4 Hold, return to the starting position, and repeat on the other side.

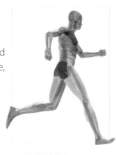

PRIMARY TARGETS

- gemellus inferior
- gemellus superior
- gluteus medius
- gluteus minimus
- piriformis
- obturator externus
- obturator internus
- pectoralis major
- pectoralis minor
- quadratus femoris
- gluteus maximus

BENEFITS

- Stretches lower back, chest, and glutes

CAUTIONS

- Severe lower-back pain

PERFECT YOUR FORM

- Keep your elbows and wrists lower than your shoulders, which will protect your rotator cuff from strain.
- Avoid lifting your shoulders; try to keep both shoulder blades in contact with the floor throughout the stretch.

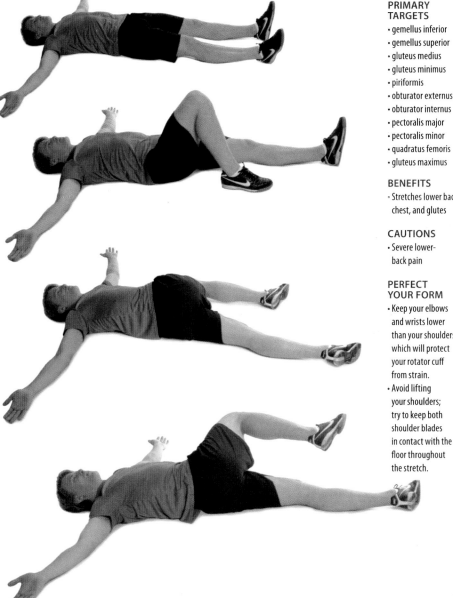

HIP/ILIOTIBIAL BAND STRETCH

INTERMEDIATE

ALL RUNNERS WANT TO KEEP their hips flexible and their iliotibial bands supple to achieve the best form and avoid running-related injury. Use the Hip/Iliotibial Band Stretch to stretch these areas while also providing yourself with a full spinal and abdominal twist.

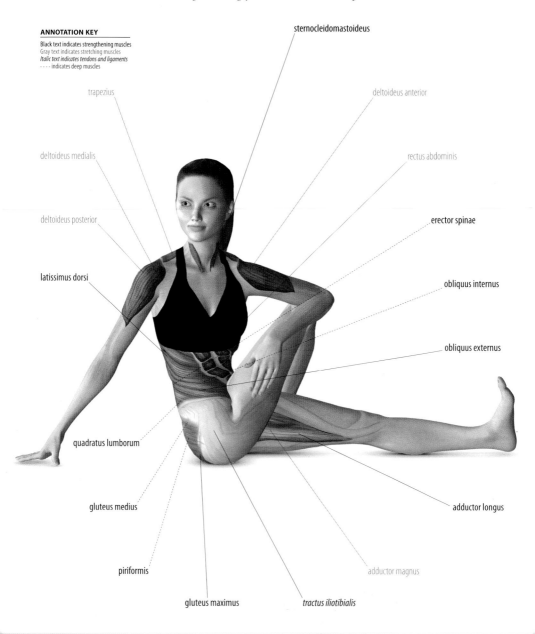

ANNOTATION KEY
Black text indicates strengthening muscles
Gray text indicates stretching muscles
Italic text indicates tendons and ligaments
- - - - indicates deep muscles

sternocleidomastoideus

trapezius

deltoideus anterior

deltoideus medialis

rectus abdominis

deltoideus posterior

erector spinae

latissimus dorsi

obliquus internus

obliquus externus

quadratus lumborum

adductor longus

gluteus medius

piriformis

adductor magnus

gluteus maximus

tractus iliotibialis

HOW TO DO IT

1 Sit on the floor, sitting up as straight as possible with your back flattened and your legs extended in front of you in parallel position. Your feet should be relaxed and flexed slightly.

2 Extend your left leg straight in front of you, and bend your right knee. Cross your bent knee over the straight leg, and keep your foot flat on the floor.

3 Wrap your left arm around the bent knee so that you are able to apply pressure to your leg to rotate your torso.

4 Keeping your hips aligned, rotate your upper spine as you pull your chest in toward your knee.

5 Hold for 30 seconds. Slowly release, and repeat three times on each side.

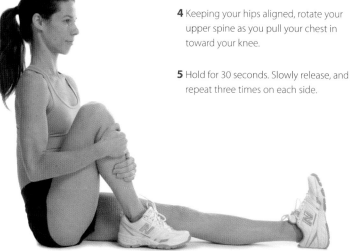

PRIMARY TARGETS

- adductor longus
- iliopsoas
- rhomboideus
- sternocleidomastoideus
- latissimus dorsi
- obliquus internus
- obliquus externus
- quadratus lumborum
- erector spinae
- multifidus spinae
- tractus iliotibialis
- gluteus maximus
- gluteus medius
- piriformis

BENEFITS

- Stretches hip extensors and flexors
- Stretches obliques

CAUTIONS

- Severe lower-back pain

PERFECT YOUR FORM

- Apply even pressure to your leg with your active hand.
- Keep your torso upright as you pull your knee and torso together.
- Avoid lifting the foot of your bent leg off the floor.

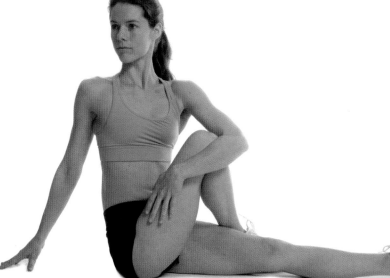

FORWARD LUNGE WITH TWIST

INTERMEDIATE

THIS VERSION OF THE FORWARD LUNGE works your glutes, thighs, and calves, just as any lunge will do, but adds a twist to bring your oblique and hip muscles into the movement, improving hip flexibility. The Forward Lunge with Twist also improves your balancing skills, which are essential for long-distance running.

ANNOTATION KEY
Black text indicates strengthening muscles
Gray text indicates stretching muscles
Italic text indicates tendons and ligaments
- - - -indicates deep muscles

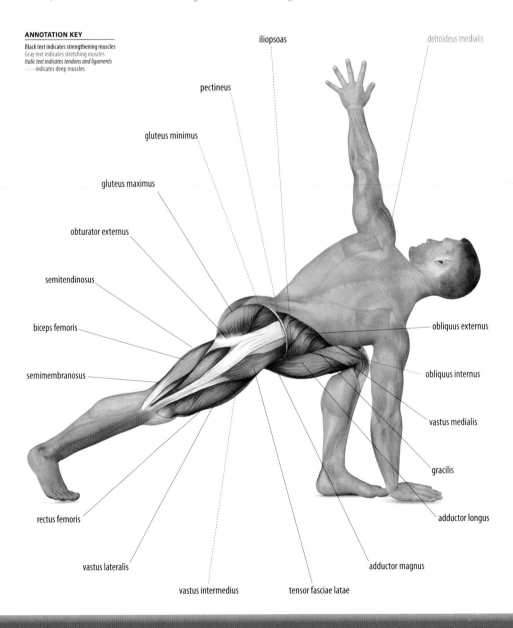

iliopsoas

deltoideus medialis

pectineus

gluteus minimus

gluteus maximus

obturator externus

semitendinosus

biceps femoris

semimembranosus

obliquus externus

obliquus internus

vastus medialis

gracilis

adductor longus

rectus femoris

adductor magnus

vastus lateralis

vastus intermedius

tensor fasciae latae

HOW TO DO IT

1 Stand with your legs and feet parallel and shoulder-width apart, and your knees bent very slightly. Tuck your pelvis slightly forward, lift your chest, and press your shoulders downward and back.

2 Bend your left knee, and step your right leg back behind your body, extending it straight.

3 Place your palms on your knee. This is the final step of Forward Lunge (see pages 34–35).

2 Fold your torso forward and place your hands on the floor on either side of your right foot.

3 Balance your weight on your left hand, and carefully and slowly guide your right arm up toward the ceiling, twisting your torso.

4 Return to the center, and repeat on the other side.

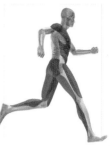

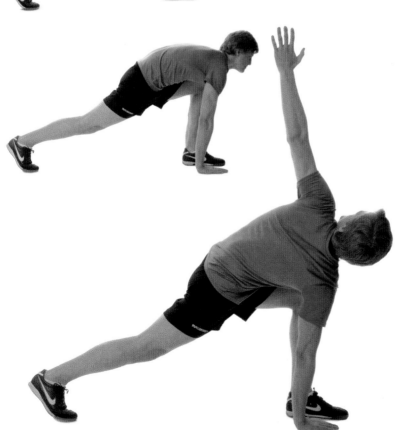

PRIMARY TARGETS

• rectus femoris
• vastus lateralis
• vastus intermedius
• vastus medialis
• biceps femoris
• semitendinosus
• semimembranosus
• gluteus minimus
• gluteus maximus
• obliquus externus
• obliquus internus
• adductor longus
• adductor magnus
• adductor brevis
• gracilis
• pectineus
• obturator externus
• iliopsoas
• tensor fasciae latae

BENEFITS

• Stretches hip flexors and core
• Strengthens glutes, hamstrings, and thighs

CAUTIONS

• Severe hip or knee degeneration

PERFECT YOUR FORM

• Keep your focus up toward your elevated arm and hand, and point the fingers of that hand in the air.
• Keep your chest slightly elevated.
• Avoid dropping the elevated arm behind you—look for both arms to remain on the same plane.

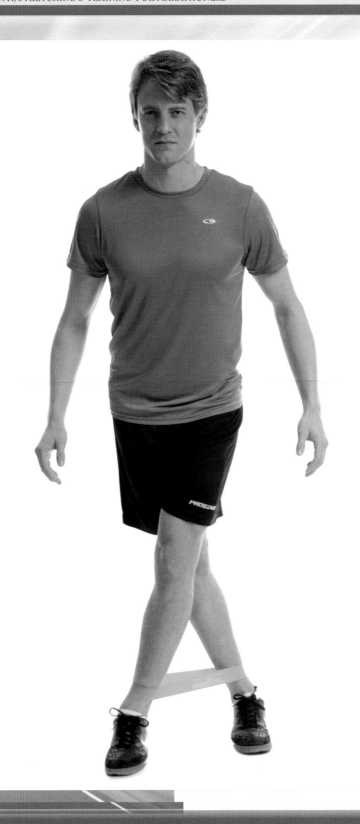

RESISTANCE BAND EXERCISES & STRETCHES

The following exercises all use resistance bands that will work your major running muscles, including those of your hips, thighs, calves, and ankles. Also known as a fitness band, Thera-Band, Dyna-Band, stretching band, and exercise band, this simple tool adds resistance to an exercise. Throughout this book, you will see two types of resistance bands: one with handles and one without. Both versions are amazing pieces of fitness equipment that effectively tone and strengthen your entire body. Bands act in a way similar to hand weights, but unlike weights, which rely on gravity to determine the resistance, bands use constant tension—supplied by your muscles—to add resistance to your movements and improve your overall coordination. Loop resistance bands are also available. These smaller elastics will add resistance to lower-leg and ankle exercises.

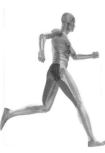

TENDON STRETCH

Achilles tendonitis afflicts many runners, so work on keeping this major tendon in good shape. Tread carefully, though, when working the Achilles tendon, making sure to avoid any excessive stretching. Instead, try a gentle stretch that also targets your posterior leg muscles, calf muscles, and hamstrings.

PRIMARY TARGETS
- tendo calcaneus
- biceps femoris
- semitendinosus
- semimembranosus
- erector spinae
- gluteus maximus
- gluteus medius
- gluteus minimus
- tendo calcaneus

BENEFITS
- Stretches Achilles tendon, lower back, hip extensors, and hip rotators

CAUTIONS
- Advanced degenerative joint disease

PERFECT YOUR FORM
- Keep even tension in both hands.
- Keep your elevated leg straight.
- Avoid lifting or bending the leg extended on the floor.

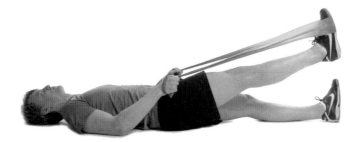

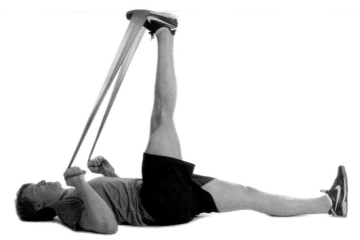

HOW TO DO IT

1 Grasp a resistance band with an end in each hand, and loop it around the bottom of your right foot. Lie on your back with your left leg extended and your spine in an imprinted position so that your lower back touches the floor. Keep your right leg elevated only high enough to maintain tension in the band.

2 Gently pull the band toward your chest with both hands so you extend and straighten your right leg toward the ceiling. Aim for a 90-degree angle, but only extend as high as is comfortable.

3 Hold for 15 to 30 seconds, switch legs, and repeat on the other side.

ANKLE STRETCHES

KEEPING YOUR ANKLES STRONG is essential if you are running—a misstep too often leads to ankle sprains, which can keep you on the sidelines, instead of in the race. These stretches work the peronei and tibialis anterior muscles that support your ankle joint.

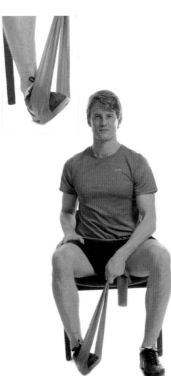
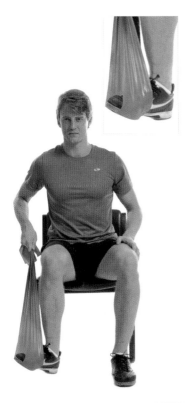

PRIMARY TARGETS
- peroneus longus
- peroneus brevis
- tibialis anterior

BENEFITS
- Stretches ankles, calves, and shins

CAUTIONS
- Acute ankle pain

PERFECT YOUR FORM
- Use a towel if you don't have an elastic resistance band.
- Avoid shifting your weight to the side while you are stretching; your weight should be evenly balanced on your sitting bones.

HOW TO DO IT

1 Sit on a chair with your back straight and your feet flat on the floor.

2 Loop an exercise band around your right foot, and then take hold of both ends of the band with your right hand.

3 Keeping your right leg stable, point your right foot and pull the band to the right, stretching the inside of your ankle.

4 Keeping the band looped around your right foot, transfer both ends of the band to your left hand.

5 Keeping your right leg stable, point your right foot and pull the band to the left, stretching the outside of your ankle.

6 Switch legs, and repeat both stretches on the other side.

ROTATION EXTENSION

AVOID THE ALL-TOO-COMMON runner's knee by keeping the muscles that support your knee in top shape. Weak or tight quadriceps often contribute to knee injury, so be sure to stretch this group of primary running muscles. This stretch targets the vastus lateralis (located on the outer thigh) and the vastus medialis (located on the inner thigh).

PRIMARY TARGETS
- vastus lateralis
- vastus medialis

BENEFITS
- Strengthens the lateral muscles of the thigh during external rotation phase of exercise
- Strengthens the medial muscles of the thigh during internal rotation phase of exercise

CAUTIONS
- Knee pain
- Ankle pain

PERFECT YOUR FORM
- Keep the thigh of the moving leg stabilized on the chair.
- Avoid lifting your knee.

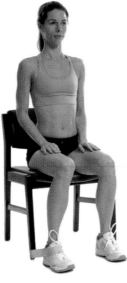

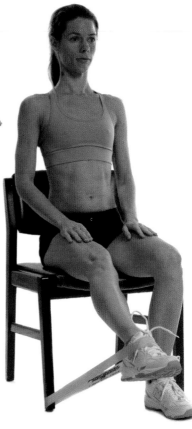

HOW TO DO IT

1 Wrap one end of an resistance band loop around a chair leg, and the other around your ankle. Sit upright on the chair, planting your feet firmly on the floor. Place your hands on your knees, and gaze forward.

2 Slowly extend and raise one leg as high as you can, or until it is parallel to the floor, with your foot flexed. Rotate it outwards, pausing at the top of the circle, and then rotate your foot inward.

3 Lower your foot, and repeat on the other side. Continue to alternate, performing two sets of 10 per side.

HIP ABDUCTION & ADDUCTION

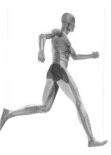

LOCATED TOWARD THE OUTSIDE portion of your thigh, the hip abductors muscles—the gluteus minimus, gluteus medius, tensor fasciae latae, and gluteus maximus—pull your thigh away from the midline of your body. Your adductors—the adductor longus, adductor magnus, adductor brevis, gracilis, pectineus, and obturator externus— are part of your inner hip and thigh musculature. Your adductors are busy muscles, pulling your leg toward the midline of your body, rotating your knee inward, dipping your pelvis downward and forward, and flexing your leg at the hip joint. Keeping these muscles strong is essential for balancing your pelvis during standing and walking.

PRIMARY TARGETS
- gluteus minimus
- gluteus medius
- tensor fasciae latae
- gluteus maximus
- adductor longus
- adductor magnus
- adductor brevis
- gracilis
- pectineus
- obturator externus

BENEFITS
- Strengthens hips

CAUTIONS
- Balance issues

PERFECT YOUR FORM
- Tighten the muscles at the side of your thigh and hip as you move your leg.
- Avoid touching your moving foot to the floor as you move your foot sideways and inward.
- Avoid leaning your torso to one side.

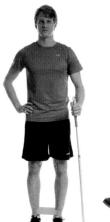
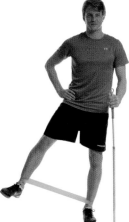
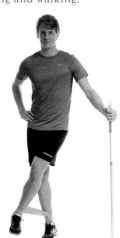

HOW TO DO IT

1 Stand with your feet shoulder-width apart, with a resistance loop or a resistance band tied around your ankles. Tuck your pelvis slightly forward, lift your chest, and press your shoulders downward and back. With your left hand, hold onto a support such as a mop handle or chair back.

2 Keeping your back and knee straight and foot facing forward, move your right foot directly to the right, moving away from your body. Hold for 2 seconds and repeat 10 times before returning to starting position.

3 Keeping your back and knee straight and foot facing forward, move your left foot directly to the right, moving it toward and across your body. Hold for 2 seconds and repeat 10 times.

5 Return to starting position, and repeat entire sequence on the opposite side.

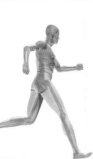

SIDE STEPS

SIDE STEPS IS A SIMPLE and fun hip-abducting exercise that gets an added boost of strengthening by incorporating the resistance band.

PRIMARY TARGETS
- gluteus minimus
- gluteus minimus
- tensor fasciae latae
- gluteus maximus

BENEFITS
- Strengthens hips

CAUTIONS
- Acute hip pain

PERFECT YOUR FORM
- Tighten the muscles at the side of your thigh and hip as you move your leg.
- Avoid leaning your torso to one side.

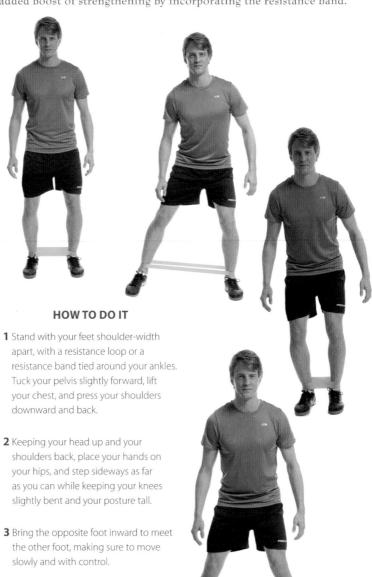

HOW TO DO IT

1 Stand with your feet shoulder-width apart, with a resistance loop or a resistance band tied around your ankles. Tuck your pelvis slightly forward, lift your chest, and press your shoulders downward and back.

2 Keeping your head up and your shoulders back, place your hands on your hips, and step sideways as far as you can while keeping your knees slightly bent and your posture tall.

3 Bring the opposite foot inward to meet the other foot, making sure to move slowly and with control.

4 Continue to step to the side for one to three sets of 8 to 12 repetitions, and then repeat in the other direction.

CROSSOVER STEPS

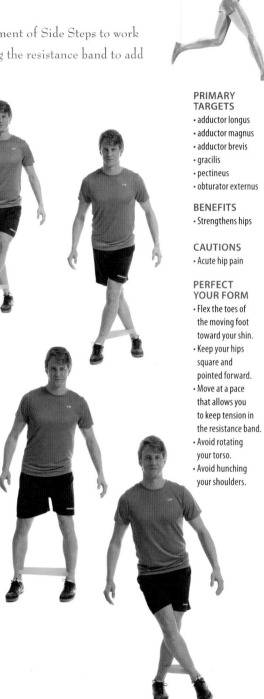

CROSSOVER STEPS reverses the movement of Side Steps to work the hip adductor muscles, again using the resistance band to add increased strengthening power.

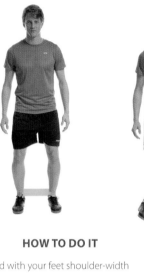

PRIMARY TARGETS
- adductor longus
- adductor magnus
- adductor brevis
- gracilis
- pectineus
- obturator externus

BENEFITS
- Strengthens hips

CAUTIONS
- Acute hip pain

PERFECT YOUR FORM
- Flex the toes of the moving foot toward your shin.
- Keep your hips square and pointed forward.
- Move at a pace that allows you to keep tension in the resistance band.
- Avoid rotating your torso.
- Avoid hunching your shoulders.

HOW TO DO IT

1 Stand with your feet shoulder-width apart, with a resistance loop or a resistance band tied around your ankles. Tuck your pelvis slightly forward, lift your chest, and press your shoulders downward and back.

2 Step out with your left foot until you feel moderate tension in the band, and then cross your left foot over your right.

3 Next, step your right foot in front of your left, and then step your left foot out, for a total of three steps with both feet to the left.

4 Return to the starting position, and then begin crossing your right foot over your left in the opposite direction.

5 Repeat all moves for a total of three sets in each direction.

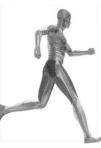

RESISTANCE BAND EXERCISES & STRETCHES

HIP EXTENSION

THE HIP EXTENSION targets your hip extensors, the muscles that pull your knee down and backward—a critical movement in running. Your gluteus maximus serves as the primary hip extensor, along with the long head of the biceps femoris, the semitendinosus, and semimembranosus.

PRIMARY TARGETS
- gluteus maximus
- biceps femoris
- semitendinosus
- semimembranosus

BENEFITS
- Strengthens hip extensor muscles

CAUTIONS
- Balance issues

PERFECT YOUR FORM
- Tighten your glutes as you move your leg backward.

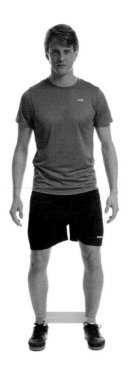

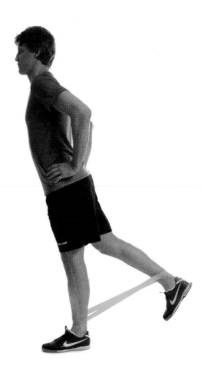

HOW TO DO IT

1 Stand with your feet shoulder-width apart, with a resistance loop or a resistance band tied around your ankles. Tuck your pelvis slightly forward, lift your chest, and press your shoulders downward and back.

2 Keeping your head up and shoulders back, place your hands on your hips, and slowly extend your leg backward.

3 Perform three sets of 10 repetitions.

If you have balance issues, hold onto a support such as a mop handle or chair back, and complete steps 1 through 3.

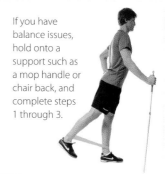

HIP FLEXION

HIP FLEXION is the movement of raising the thigh upward—another important running movement. The iliopsoas is the main hip flexor, along with the rectus femoris and sartorius. Performing the Hip Flexion exercise with a resistance band strengthens these muscles.

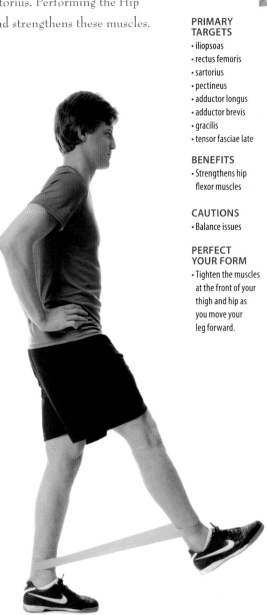

PRIMARY TARGETS
- iliopsoas
- rectus femoris
- sartorius
- pectineus
- adductor longus
- adductor brevis
- gracilis
- tensor fasciae late

BENEFITS
- Strengthens hip flexor muscles

CAUTIONS
- Balance issues

PERFECT YOUR FORM
- Tighten the muscles at the front of your thigh and hip as you move your leg forward.

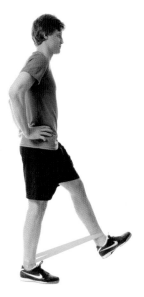

HOW TO DO IT

1 Stand with your feet shoulder-width apart, with a resistance loop or a resistance band tied around your ankles. Tuck your pelvis slightly forward, lift your chest, and press your shoulders downward and back.

2 Keeping your back and knee straight, slowly extend your left leg forward.

3 Return to starting position, and extend forward again, performing three sets of 10 repetitions.

4 Return to starting position, and repeat entire sequence on the opposite side.

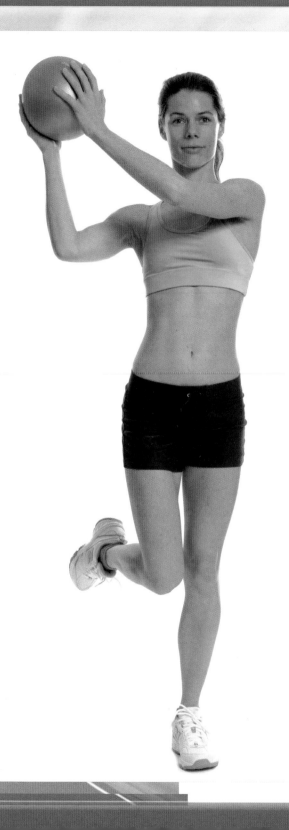

TRAINING YOUR PRIMARY MUSCLES

Whether your run a marathon or just jog around the local park, as you run, your body primarily calls on a few large muscle groups: your quadriceps, hamstrings, gluteals, and iliopsoas. The large quadriceps femoris group, made up of the rectus femoris, vastus lateralis, vastus intermedius, and vastus medialis, is located at the front of the thigh; located on the back of the thigh, the biceps femoris, semitendinosus, and semimembranosus make up the group known as the hamstrings. The largest muscle in your body—the gluteus maximus—really comes into play only when you run, along with the gluteus medius and gluteus minimus. The last of the primary running muscles is the iliopsoas (also known as the psoas major and iliacus).

The following exercises target these large antagonist and agonist muscles, which work in concert to move and stabilize you. An antagonist pair consists of an extensor muscle, such as the gluteus maximus, which "opens" the hip joint, and a flexor, such as the iliopsoas, which does the opposite. Keeping them in proper balance (size, strength, and elasticity) is crucial to avoid running-related injuries and increase your performance levels.

To aid you while performing the exercises in your running routine, take advantage of everyday objects around the house: grasp a mop handle for balance or use steps for lunges and calf exercises. Many of the featured exercises incorporate equipment, such as hand weights, dumbbells, and medicine balls, which add variety and challenge to your workout. Also featured are Swiss ball exercises. This heavy-duty inflatable ball comes in a variety of sizes. Be sure to find the best size for your height and weight (when you sit on the ball, your thighs should be parallel or slightly above parallel to the floor). Its instability makes it an excellent fitness tool: you must constantly adjust your balance while performing a movement, which helps you improve your overall sense of balance and your flexibility.

KNEE SQUAT

BEGINNER

The Knee Squat integrates balance, coordination, resistance, and stretching to target your leg muscles. This exercise also strengthens the muscles of your feet.

ANNOTATION KEY

Black text indicates strengthening muscles
Gray text indicates stretching muscles
Italic text indicates tendons and ligaments
---- indicates deep muscles

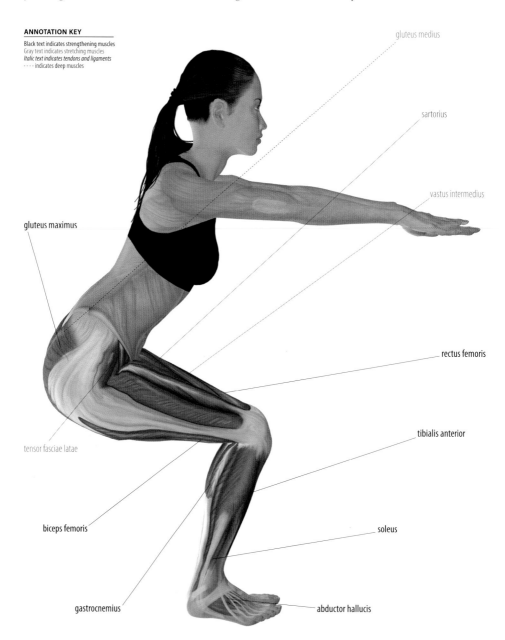

gluteus medius

sartorius

vastus intermedius

gluteus maximus

rectus femoris

tibialis anterior

tensor fasciae latae

biceps femoris

soleus

gastrocnemius

abductor hallucis

HOW TO DO IT

1 Stand with your legs and feet parallel and shoulder-width apart, and your knees bent very slightly. Tuck your pelvis slightly forward, lift your chest, and press your shoulders downward and back.

2 Extend your arms in front of your body for stability, keeping them even with your shoulders. Plant your feet firmly on the floor, and curl your toes slightly upward.

3 Draw in your abdominal muscles and bend into a squat. Keep your heels planted on the floor and your chest as upright as possible, resisting the urge to bend too far forward.

4 Exhale, and return to the original position. Repeat five to six times.

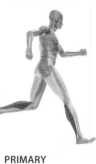

PRIMARY TARGETS

• biceps femoris
• rectus femoris
• tibialis anterior
• gastrocnemius
• soleus
• gluteus maximus
• abductor hallucis
• vastus medialis

BENEFITS

• Lengthens and strengthens calf muscles
• Improves balance

CAUTIONS

• Foot pain

PERFECT YOUR FORM

• Keep your chest upright.
• Pull your abdominals in toward your spine.
• Curl your toes upward throughout the movement.
• Imagine pressing into the floor as you rise from the squat, creating your body's own resistance in your leg muscles.
• Avoid allowing your heels to lift off the floor.
• Avoid rising too quickly to the standing position.

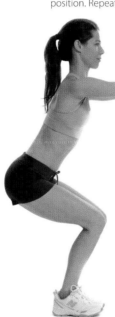

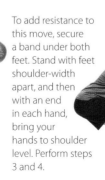

Challenge yourself by adding weight to this exercise by grasping a weighted medicine ball in both hands, and then following steps 1 though 4.

To add resistance to this move, secure a band under both feet. Stand with feet shoulder-width apart, and then with an end in each hand, bring your hands to shoulder level. Perform steps 3 and 4.

LATERAL LOW LUNGE

BEGINNER

THE LATERAL LOW LUNGE, also known as a Side Lunge, increases the mobility of your hips and loosens the muscles of your glutes and groins while opening up your calves, quads, hamstrings, lateral thighs, and hips.

ANNOTATION KEY
Black text indicates strengthening muscles
Gray text indicates stretching muscles
Italic text indicates tendons and ligaments
- - - - indicates deep muscles

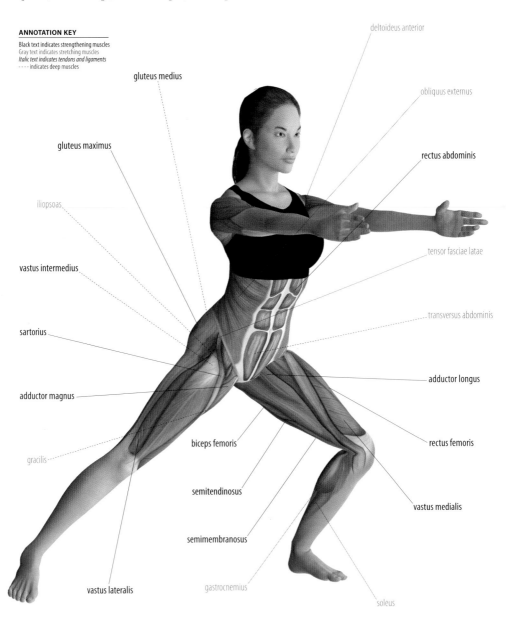

gluteus medius

gluteus maximus

iliopsoas

vastus intermedius

sartorius

adductor magnus

gracilis

vastus lateralis

biceps femoris

semitendinosus

semimembranosus

gastrocnemius

deltoideus anterior

obliquus externus

rectus abdominis

tensor fasciae latae

transversus abdominis

adductor longus

rectus femoris

vastus medialis

soleus

HOW TO DO IT

1 Stand with your feet planted widely and your arms outstretched in front of you, parallel to the floor.

2 Step out to the left. Squat down on your left leg, bending at your hips, while maintaining a neutral spine. Begin to extend your right leg, keeping both feet flat on the floor.

3 Bend your left knee until your thigh is parallel to the floor, and your right leg is fully extended.

4 Keeping your arms parallel to the floor, squeeze your buttocks and press off your left leg to return to the starting position, and repeat. Repeat sequence 10 times on each side.

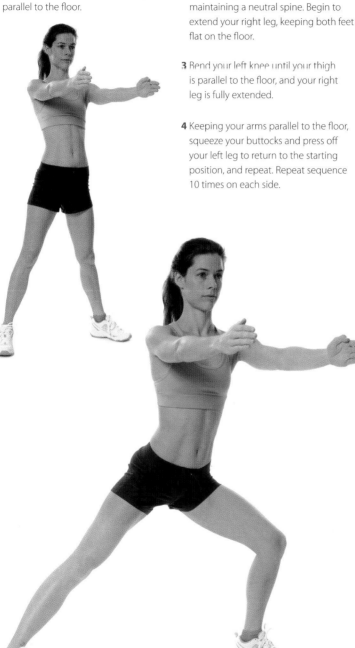

PRIMARY TARGETS
- adductor longus
- adductor magnus
- semitendinosus
- semimembranosus
- biceps femoris
- sartorius
- vastus medialis
- vastus lateralis
- vastus intermedius
- rectus femoris
- gluteus maximus
- gluteus medius
- rectus abdominis

BENEFITS
- Strengthens the trunk, knee, and pelvic stabilizers

CAUTIONS
- Knee pain
- Back pain
- Trouble bearing weight on one leg

PERFECT YOUR FORM
- Keep your spine in neutral position as you bend your hips.
- Relax your neck and shoulders.
- Align your knee with the toe of your bent leg.
- Tighten your glutes as you bend.
- Avoid craning your neck as you perform the movement.
- Avoid lifting your feet off the floor.
- Avoid arching or extending your back.

STEP-DOWN

BEGINNER

STEP-DOWN is a great strength builder for the muscles that support your knees and pelvis. Regularly performing it will improve knee control and strengthen your quads for downhill running, while also improving your balance and core strength.

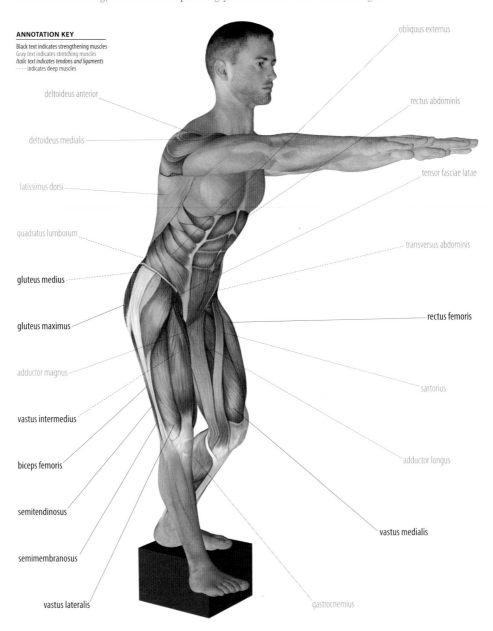

ANNOTATION KEY
Black text indicates strengthening muscles
Gray text indicates stretching muscles
Italic text indicates tendons and ligaments
---- indicates deep muscles

deltoideus anterior

deltoideus medialis

latissimus dorsi

quadratus lumborum

gluteus medius

gluteus maximus

adductor magnus

vastus intermedius

biceps femoris

semitendinosus

semimembranosus

vastus lateralis

obliquus externus

rectus abdominis

tensor fasciae latae

transversus abdominis

rectus femoris

sartorius

adductor longus

vastus medialis

gastrocnemius

HOW TO DO IT

1 Standing up straight on a firm step or block, firmly plant your left foot close to the edge, allowing your right foot to hang off the side. Flex the toes of your right foot.

2 Lift your arms out in front of you for balance, keeping them parallel to the floor. Lower your torso as you bend at your hips and knees, dropping your right leg toward the floor.

3 Without rotating your torso or knee, press upward through your left leg to return to the starting position. Repeat 15 times for two sets on each leg.

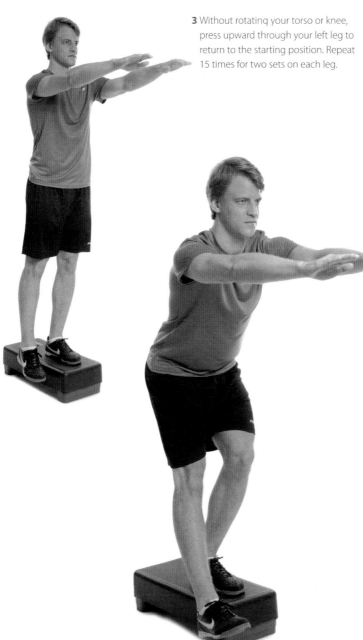

PRIMARY TARGETS
- vastus medialis
- vastus lateralis
- vastus intermedius
- rectus femoris
- gluteus maximus
- gluteus medius
- semitendinosus
- semimembranosus
- biceps femoris

BENEFITS
- Strengthens pelvic and knee stabilizers

CAUTIONS
- Ankle pain
- Sharp knee pain
- Lower-back pain

PERFECT YOUR FORM
- Align your bent knee with your second toe so that your knee doesn't rotate inward.
- Bend your knees and hips at the same time.
- Keep your hips behind your foot, leaning your torso forward as you lower into the bend.
- Avoid craning your neck.
- Avoid placing weight on the foot being lowered to the floor—only allow a touch.

YOGA LUNGE

BEGINNER

THIS VERSION OF A FORWARD LUNGE is usually called High Lunge in yoga, but it is also known as a low forward lunge. It is an effective leg and arm strengthener that targets your glutes and quadriceps, along with your hamstrings, soleus, and gastrocnemius muscles. The deep position will also stretch your groins.

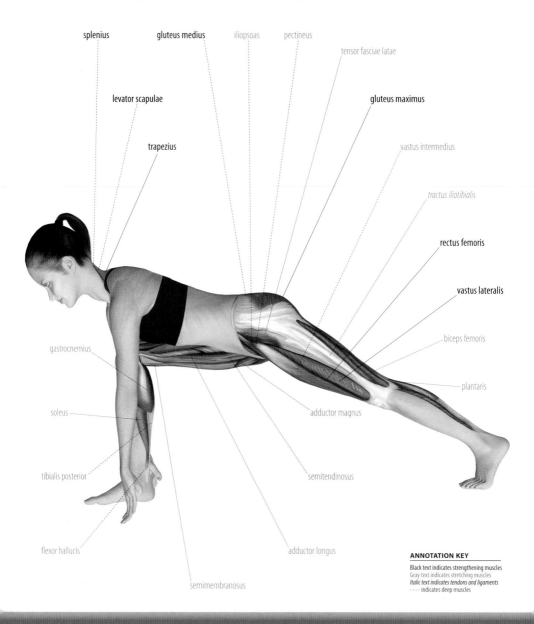

splenius

gluteus medius

iliopsoas

pectineus

tensor fasciae latae

levator scapulae

gluteus maximus

vastus intermedius

trapezius

tractus iliotibialis

rectus femoris

vastus lateralis

gastrocnemius

biceps femoris

soleus

plantaris

adductor magnus

tibialis posterior

semitendinosus

flexor hallucis

adductor longus

semimembranosus

ANNOTATION KEY

Black text indicates strengthening muscles
Gray text indicates stretching muscles
Italic text indicates tendons and ligaments
- - - - indicates deep muscles

HOW TO DO IT

1 Stand with your feet together and your arms hanging at your sides.

2 Exhale, and carefully step back with your left leg, keeping it in line with your hips as you step back. The ball of your right foot should be in contact with the floor as you do the motion.

3 Slowly slide your left foot farther back while bending your right knee, stacking it directly above your ankle.

4 Position your palms or fingertips on the floor on either side of your right leg, and slowly press your palms or fingertips against the floor to enhance the placement of your upper body and your head.

5 Lift your head and gaze straight forward while leaning your upper body forward and carefully rolling your shoulders downward and back.

6 Press the ball of your right foot gradually into the floor, contract your thigh muscles, and press up to keep your left leg straight.

7 Hold for 5 seconds. Slowly return to the starting position, and then repeat on the other side.

TRAINING YOUR PRIMARY MUSCLES

PRIMARY TARGETS
- biceps femoris
- adductor longus
- adductor magnus
- gastrocnemius
- tibialis posterior
- iliopsoas
- biceps femoris
- rectus femoris

BENEFITS
- Strengthens legs and arms
- Stretches groins

CAUTIONS
- Arm injury
- Shoulder injury
- Hip injury
- High or low blood pressure
- Severe headache

PERFECT YOUR FORM
- Maintain proper position of your shoulders and your whole upper body to lengthen your spine.
- Avoid dropping your back-extended knee to the floor.

DUMBBELL DEADLIFT

INTERMEDIATE

THE DEADLIFT is a weight-training exercise in which you lift weight off the ground from a stabilized, bent-over position. It is a compound movement that primarily works the gluteus maximus and hamstrings to extend your hip joints, the quadriceps to extend your knee joints, and the adductor magnus to stabilize your legs.

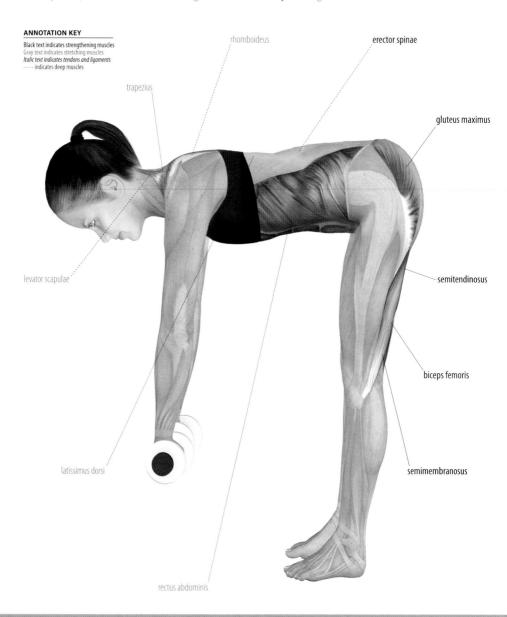

ANNOTATION KEY
Black text indicates strengthening muscles
Gray text indicates stretching muscles
Italic text indicates tendons and ligaments
- - - - indicates deep muscles

rhomboideus

erector spinae

trapezius

gluteus maximus

levator scapulae

semitendinosus

biceps femoris

latissimus dorsi

semimembranosus

rectus abdominis

HOW TO DO IT

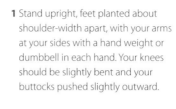

1 Stand upright, feet planted about shoulder-width apart, with your arms at your sides with a hand weight or dumbbell in each hand. Your knees should be slightly bent and your buttocks pushed slightly outward.

2 Keeping your back flat, hinge at the hips and bend forward as you lower the dumbbells toward the floor. You should feel a stretch in the backs of your legs.

3 With control, raise your upper body back to starting position. Repeat, completing three sets of 15.

PRIMARY TARGETS
- biceps femoris
- semitendinosus
- semimembranosus
- erector spinae
- gluteus maximus

BENEFITS
- Improves flexibility
- Stabilizes lower body

CAUTIONS
- Lower-back pain

PERFECT YOUR FORM
- Maintain the straight line of your back.
- Keep your torso stable.
- Keep your neck straight.
- Keep your arms extended.
- Avoid allowing your lower back to sag or arch.
- Avoid straining to look forward while you are bent over.

TRAINING YOUR PRIMARY MUSCLES

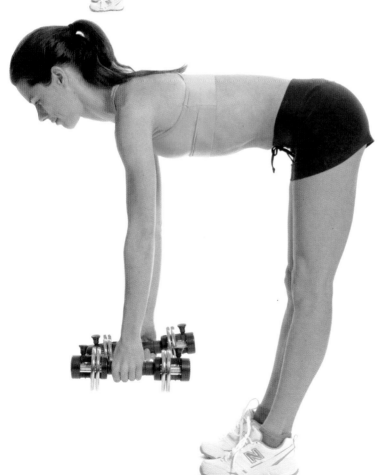

RESISTANCE BAND LUNGE

INTERMEDIATE

By ADDING A RESISTANCE BAND, you make a lunge a more challenging movement as you work your lower body. The Resistance Band Lunge can be incorporated into deceleration training, which prepares your body to take on a load in the negative aspect of a movement, such as coming to a stop after running. This improves your ability to absorb the acceleration phase of a running stride and enhances your form.

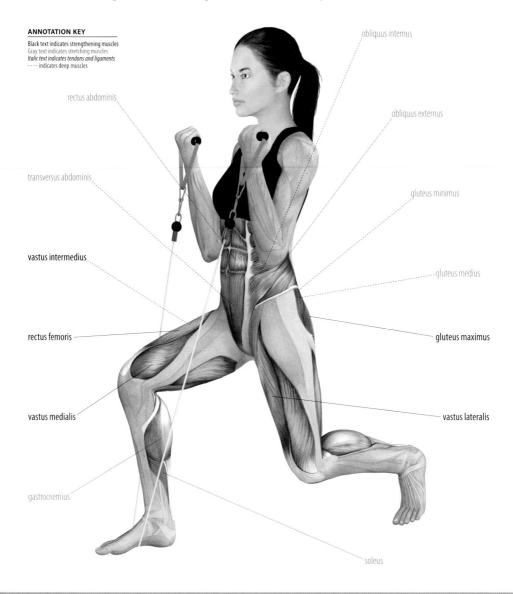

ANNOTATION KEY
Black text indicates strengthening muscles
Gray text indicates stretching muscles
Italic text indicates tendons and ligaments
- - - - indicates deep muscles

obliquus internus

rectus abdominis

obliquus externus

transversus abdominis

gluteus minimus

vastus intermedius

gluteus medius

rectus femoris

gluteus maximus

vastus medialis

vastus lateralis

gastrocnemius

soleus

HOW TO DO IT

1 Position a resistance band beneath your right foot, grasping both handles.

2 Keeping your head up and your spine neutral, take a big step forward.

3 Drop your left knee toward the floor, bending both legs until your right thigh is parallel to the ground. At the same time, bring the resistance band closer to your body with palms facing your shoulders.

4 Slowly and with control, straighten your legs as you raise your body, and return your arms to starting position. Complete 15 repetitions, switch sides, and repeat for three sets of 15 on each leg.

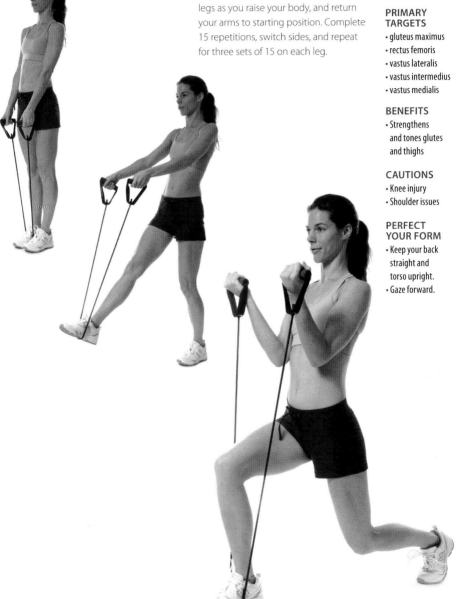

PRIMARY TARGETS
• gluteus maximus
• rectus femoris
• vastus lateralis
• vastus intermedius
• vastus medialis

BENEFITS
• Strengthens and tones glutes and thighs

CAUTIONS
• Knee injury
• Shoulder issues

PERFECT YOUR FORM
• Keep your back straight and torso upright.
• Gaze forward.

TRAINING YOUR PRIMARY MUSCLES

DUMBBELL LUNGE

INTERMEDIATE

WITH ALL THE BENEFITS of the Resistance Band Lunge, a weighted lunge, such as the Dumbbell Lunge, adds additional muscle work to a forward lunge, and introduces a weight-bearing element, which is vital to your bone health.

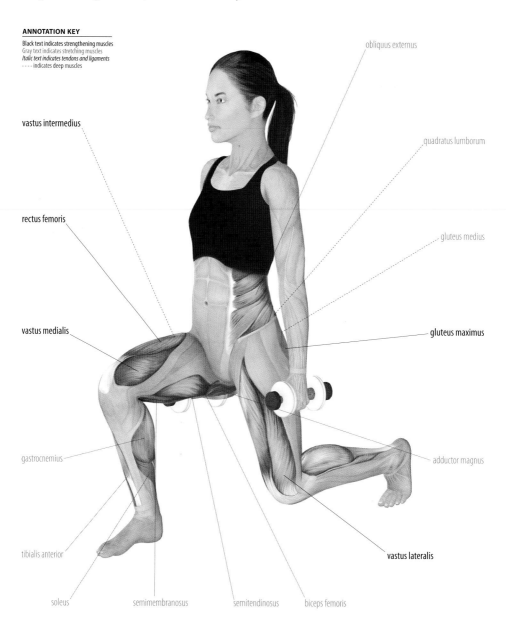

ANNOTATION KEY
Black text indicates strengthening muscles
Gray text indicates stretching muscles
Italic text indicates tendons and ligaments
- - - - indicates deep muscles

vastus intermedius

rectus femoris

vastus medialis

gastrocnemius

tibialis anterior

soleus

semimembranosus

semitendinosus

biceps femoris

obliquus externus

quadratus lumborum

gluteus medius

gluteus maximus

adductor magnus

vastus lateralis

HOW TO DO IT

1 Stand with your feet planted about shoulder-width apart, with your arms at your sides and a hand weight or dumbbell in each hand.

2 Keeping your head up and your spine neutral, take a big step forward on your right foot.

3 In one movement as you step forward, bend your right knee to a 90-degree angle, dropping your thigh until it is parallel to the floor. Your left knee will drop behind you so that you are balancing on the toe of your left foot, creating a straight line from your spine to the back of your knee.

3 Push through your right heel to stand upright, and then return to starting position. Repeat on the other leg, alternating to perform three sets of 15 lunges per leg.

PRIMARY TARGETS
- gluteus maximus
- rectus femoris
- vastus lateralis
- vastus intermedius
- vastus medialis

BENEFITS
- Strengthens and tones quadriceps and glutes

CAUTIONS
- Knee issues

PERFECT YOUR FORM
- Keep your body facing forward as you step one leg in front of you.
- Stand upright.
- Gaze forward.
- Ease into the lunge.
- Make sure that your front knee is facing forward.
- Avoid turning your body to one side.
- Avoid allowing your knee to extend past your foot.
- Avoid arching your back.

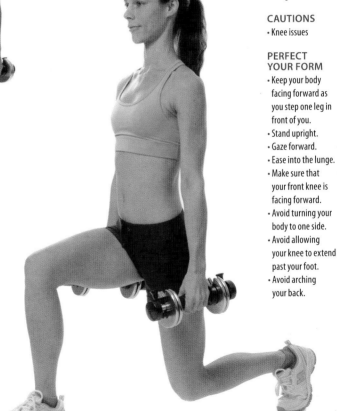

WALL SIT

INTERMEDIATE

THE WALL SIT is an excellent isometric exercise that targets the all-important quads, glutes, and calves. In an isometric exercise, the contracting muscles produce little or no movement, but you'll gain leg strength and endurance for long-distance running.

ANNOTATION KEY

Black text indicates strengthening muscles
Gray text indicates stretching muscles
Italic text indicates tendons and ligaments
---- indicates deep muscles

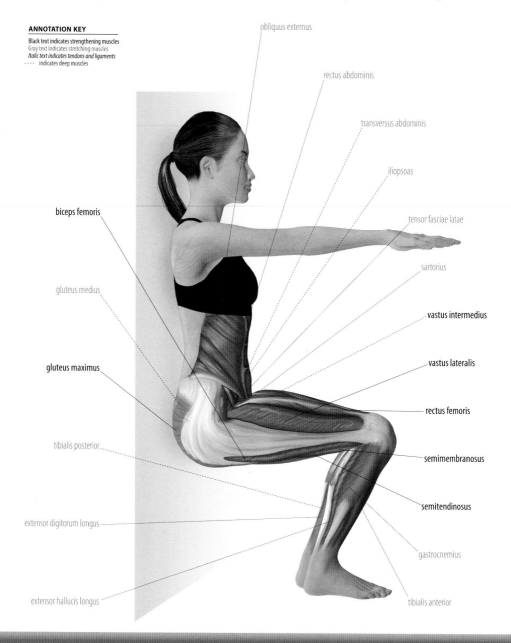

obliquus externus

rectus abdominis

transversus abdominis

iliopsoas

tensor fasciae latae

sartorius

vastus intermedius

vastus lateralis

rectus femoris

semimembranosus

semitendinosus

gastrocnemius

tibialis anterior

biceps femoris

gluteus medius

gluteus maximus

tibialis posterior

extensor digitorum longus

extensor hallucis longus

HOW TO DO IT

1 Stand with your back to a wall. Lean against the wall, and walk your feet out from under your body until your lower back rests comfortably against it.

2 Slide your torso down the wall, until your hips and knees form 90-degree angles, your thighs parallel to the floor.

3 Raise your arms straight in front of you so that they are parallel to your thighs, and relax your upper torso. Hold for 1 minute, and repeat five times.

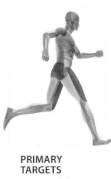

PRIMARY TARGETS

- vastus medialis
- vastus lateralis
- vastus intermedius
- rectus femoris
- semitendinosus
- semimembranosus
- biceps femoris
- gluteus maximus

BENEFITS

- Strengthens quadriceps and gluteal muscles
- Trains the body to place weight evenly between the legs

CAUTIONS

- Knee pain

PERFECT YOUR FORM

- Keep your body firm throughout the exercise.
- Relax your neck and shoulders.
- Form a 90-degree angle with your hips and knees to receive maximum benefit from the exercise.
- Avoid sitting below 90 degrees.
- Don't push your back into the wall to hold yourself up.
- Avoid shifting from side to side as you begin to fatigue.

SWISS BALL WALL SQUATS

INTERMEDIATE

SWISS BALL WALL SQUATS, unlike the isometric Wall Sit, is a dynamic exercise involving concentric and eccentric contractions of your quads and hamstrings. It provides an intense workout that will help you increase your speed and build your endurance.

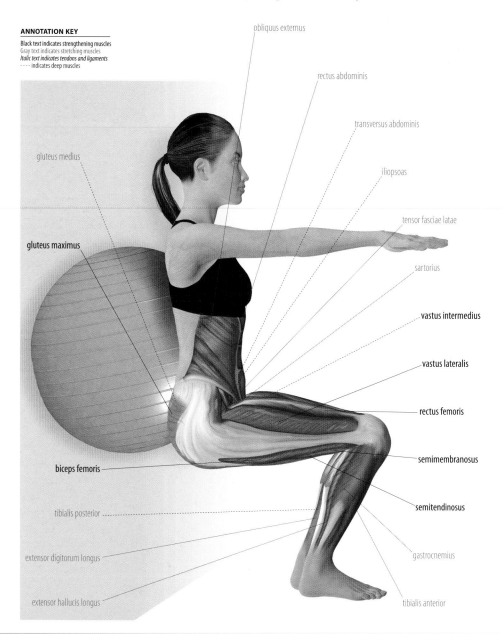

ANNOTATION KEY

Black text indicates strengthening muscles
Gray text indicates stretching muscles
Italic text indicates tendons and ligaments
- - - - indicates deep muscles

obliquus externus

rectus abdominis

transversus abdominis

iliopsoas

tensor fasciae latae

sartorius

vastus intermedius

vastus lateralis

rectus femoris

semimembranosus

semitendinosus

gastrocnemius

tibialis anterior

gluteus medius

gluteus maximus

biceps femoris

tibialis posterior

extensor digitorum longus

extensor hallucis longus

HOW TO DO IT

1 Place a Swiss ball against a wall and stand with your back to it so that your back and shoulders are pinning it to the wall. Your feet should be about hip-width apart, but slightly ahead of your hips.

2 Raise your arms straight in front of you so that they are parallel to your thighs, and relax your upper torso.

3 Keeping the ball pinned against the wall, slowly bend your hips and knees as you lower to a sitting position, rolling the ball down the wall with you as you sit.

4 Hold for a count of 10, and then press back upward to the starting position, rolling the ball up the wall with your shoulders as you rise. Repeat for a second set of 10.

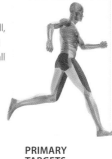

TRAINING YOUR PRIMARY MUSCLES

PRIMARY TARGETS
- vastus medialis
- vastus lateralis
- vastus intermedius
- rectus femoris
- semitendinosus
- semimembranosus
- biceps femoris
- gluteus maximus

BENEFITS
- Strengthens quadriceps and gluteal muscles
- Trains the body to place weight evenly between the legs

CAUTIONS
- Knee pain

PERFECT YOUR FORM
- Place your feet ahead of your hips by half the length of your thigh.
- Keep your body firm throughout the exercise.
- Relax your neck and shoulders.
- Avoid dipping below 90 degrees.

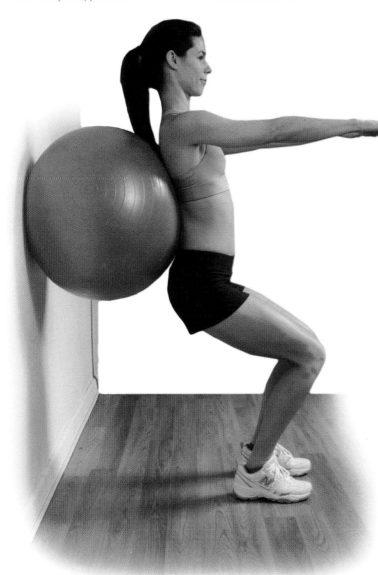

SWISS BALL LOOP EXTENSION

INTERMEDIATE

THE SWISS BALL LOOP EXTENSION challenges your balance and strength, calling for you to remain stable on the ball in plank position while extending your legs upward against the resistance of the loop band. It not only works the glutes and hamstrings, but also tightens and tones your abdominal muscles.

ANNOTATION KEY

Black text indicates strengthening muscles
Gray text indicates stretching muscles
Italic text indicates tendons and ligaments
- - - - indicates deep muscles

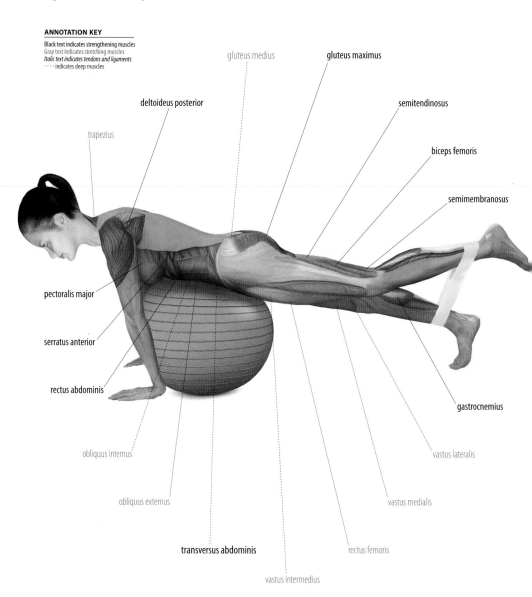

gluteus medius

gluteus maximus

deltoideus posterior

semitendinosus

trapezius

biceps femoris

semimembranosus

pectoralis major

serratus anterior

rectus abdominis

gastrocnemius

obliquus internus

vastus lateralis

obliquus externus

vastus medialis

transversus abdominis

rectus femoris

vastus intermedius

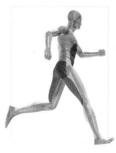

HOW TO DO IT

1 With a resistance band tied around your ankles, lie prone on a Swiss ball, with your hips over the center of the ball as you support your weight on your arms. Your hands should be directly below your shoulders.

2 Keeping your abs tight, exhale, and squeeze your glutes to raise your right leg, lengthening your body as your weight transfers from your arms to your left foot, stretching through your heel.

3 Return your right foot to the floor. Repeat 10 leg extensions on that side, holding a straight plank position throughout the exercise.

4 Switch legs, and repeat 10 times on the other side.

PRIMARY TARGETS

- gluteus maximus
- biceps femoris
- semitendinosus
- semimembranosus
- pectoralis major
- serratus anterior
- deltoideus posterior
- rectus abdominis
- transversus abdominis
- gastrocnemius

BENEFITS

- Strengthens hips and hamstrings
- Strengthens abs

CAUTIONS

- Shoulder issues

PERFECT YOUR FORM

- Keep your hips in line with your shoulders and ankles to achieve optimal weight distribution.
- Keep your neck elongated and relaxed.
- Keep your core tight and your back flat.
- Avoid allowing your shoulders to sink.

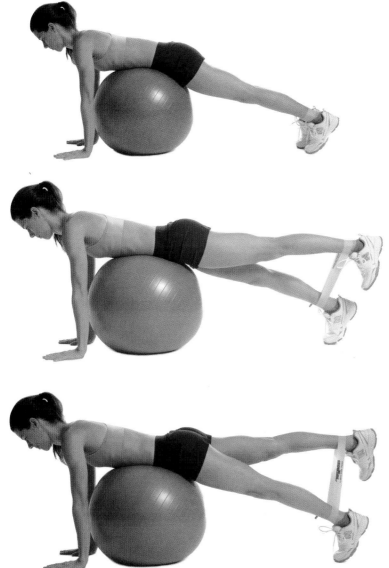

PLANK LEG EXTENSION

ADVANCED

THE PLANK LEG EXTENSION takes the basic isometric plank exercise, which works to stabilize your core and strengthen your shoulders, arms, and back, and adds a dynamic element that will target your glutes and hamstrings. It requires you to possess a high level of balance and control over your arms and legs. During the leg extension portion of the exercise, your spine should "float" over your body.

ANNOTATION KEY
Black text indicates strengthening muscles
Gray text indicates stretching muscles
Italic text indicates tendons and ligaments
- - - - indicates deep muscles

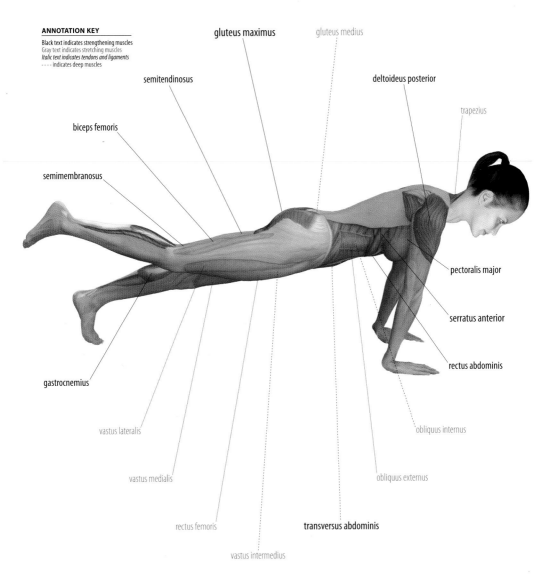

gluteus maximus

gluteus medius

semitendinosus

deltoideus posterior

trapezius

biceps femoris

semimembranosus

pectoralis major

serratus anterior

rectus abdominis

gastrocnemius

vastus lateralis

obliquus internus

vastus medialis

obliquus externus

rectus femoris

transversus abdominis

vastus intermedius

TRAINING YOUR PRIMARY MUSCLES

HOW TO DO IT

1 In prone position, support your upper body with your hands, your arms straight below your shoulders. Your legs should be straight and hip-width apart.

2 Keeping your abs tight, exhale, and squeeze your glutes to raise your right leg, lengthening your body as your weight transfers from your arms to your left foot, stretching through your heel.

3 Return your right foot to the floor. Repeat 10 leg extensions on that side, holding a straight plank position throughout the exercise.

4 Switch legs, and repeat 10 times on the other side.

PRIMARY TARGETS
- gluteus maximus
- pectoralis major
- serratus anterior
- deltoideus posterior
- rectus abdominis
- biceps femoris
- semitendinosus
- semimembranosus
- transversus abdominis
- obliquus externus

BENEFITS
- Strengthens abs
- Strengthens hips and hamstrings
- Stabilizes the spine against gravity

CAUTIONS
- Shoulder issues

PERFECT YOUR FORM
- Keep your hips in line with your shoulders and ankles to achieve optimal weight distribution.
- Keep your neck elongated and relaxed.
- Don't allow your lower back to sag as you fatigue.

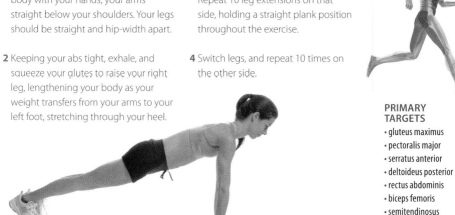

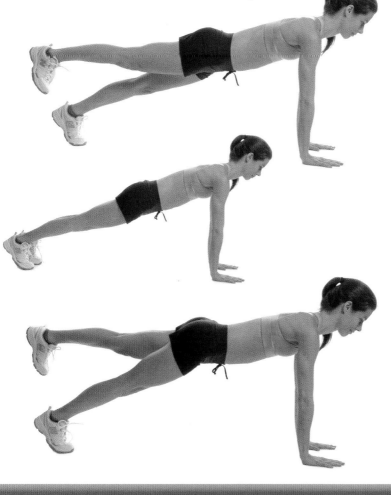

POWER SQUAT

ADVANCED

POWER SQUAT OFFERS a full-body workout that develops coordination and balance. With the benefits of both a squat and a deadlift to strengthen and tone your thighs and calves, it also calls for spinal rotation that works your back and obliques.

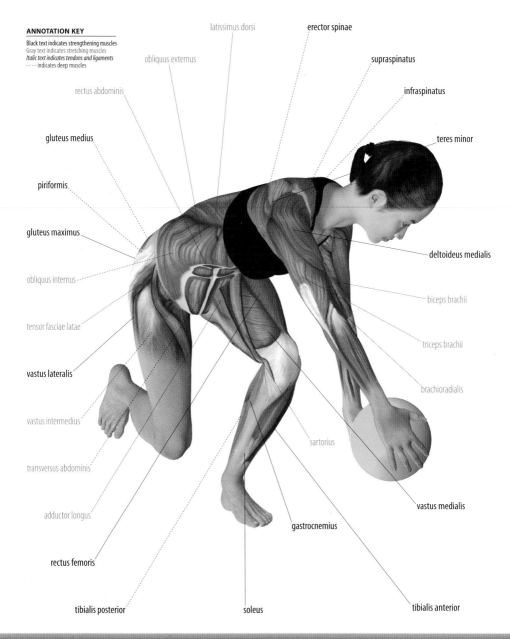

ANNOTATION KEY
Black text indicates strengthening muscles
Gray text indicates stretching muscles
Italic text indicates tendons and ligaments
- - - - indicates deep muscles

latissimus dorsi

erector spinae

obliquus externus

supraspinatus

infraspinatus

rectus abdominis

teres minor

gluteus medius

piriformis

gluteus maximus

deltoideus medialis

obliquus internus

biceps brachii

tensor fasciae latae

triceps brachii

vastus lateralis

brachioradialis

vastus intermedius

transversus abdominis

sartorius

adductor longus

vastus medialis

rectus femoris

gastrocnemius

tibialis posterior

soleus

tibialis anterior

HOW TO DO IT

1 Stand straight, holding a weighted medicine ball in front of your torso.

2 Shift your weight to your left foot, and bend your right knee, lifting your right foot toward your buttocks. Bend your elbows and draw the ball toward the outside of your right ear.

3 Maintaining a neutral spine, bend at your hips and knee. Lower your torso toward your left side, bringing the ball toward your left ankle.

4 Press into your left leg and straighten your knee and torso, returning to the starting position. Repeat 15 times for two sets on each leg.

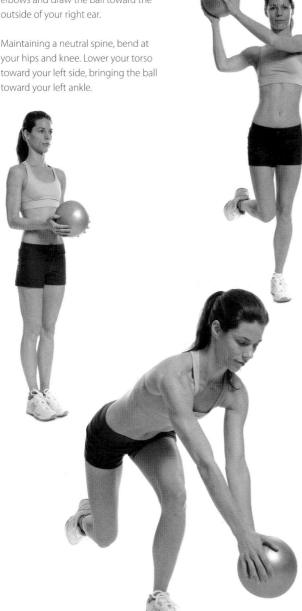

TRAINING YOUR PRIMARY MUSCLES

PRIMARY TARGETS

- vastus medialis
- vastus lateralis
- rectus femoris
- gluteus maximus
- gluteus medius
- piriformis
- erector spinae
- tibialis anterior
- tibialis posterior
- soleus
- gastrocnemius
- deltoideus medialis
- infraspinatus
- supraspinatus
- teres minor
- semitendinosus
- semimembranosus
- biceps femoris

BENEFITS

- Improves balance
- Stabilizes pelvis, trunk, and knees
- Promotes stronger movement patterns

CAUTIONS

- Knee pain
- Lower-back pain
- Shoulder pain

PERFECT YOUR FORM

- Keep your leading knee tight.
- Avoid allowing your knee to extend beyond your toes as you bend and rotate.
- Avoid moving your standing foot from its starting position.
- Move the ball in an arc through the air.

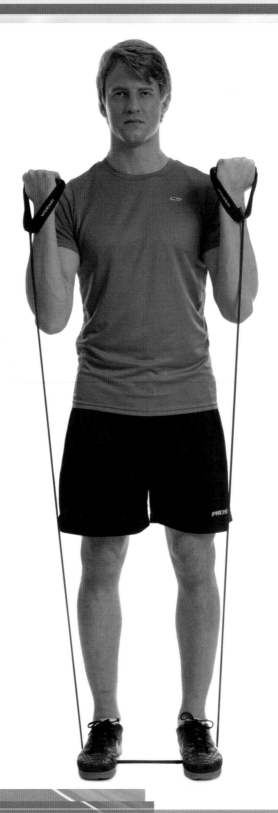

TRAINING YOUR SECONDARY MUSCLES

Running demands that your entire body work hard, including your core, back, shoulders, and arms. Building strength in these secondary areas will help you run more efficiently, with greater endurance and a lowered risk of injury.

Your core is made up of the deep muscle layers that lie close to the spine, including the abdominals (rectus abdominis, transversus abdominis, obliquus externus, and obliquus internus), the spinal extensors (multifidus spinae, erector spinae, splenius, and semispinalis) and the diaphragm. During a run, it stabilizes your trunk and pelvis, allowing your arms and legs to move properly. Working on the minor core muscles, such as the latissimus dorsi (the large smooth muscle of your back) and the trapezius (the triangle-shaped muscle on the upper back and neck), will also help you run better and strengthen your back.

When devising your marathon training regimen, don't forget the arms and shoulders, which must pump effectively to keep you balanced as you move. Included here are exercises that target these muscles too, including the deltoids, biceps, and triceps.

Also included are exercises featuring a foam roller. Rollers come in a variety of sizes, materials, and densities, and they can be used for stretching, strengthening, balance training, stability training, and self-massage. If you do not have access to a foam roller, you can substitute a swimming noodle or a homemade towel roller. To make a towel roller, place two bath towels together, firmly roll them lengthwise, and then wrap the ends with tape. Although a towel roller works well, the dense foam of the roller will provide you with the best results.

UNILATERAL LEG CIRCLES

BEGINNER

ONE OF THE BASIC EXERCISES of Pilates, Unilateral Leg Circles are an effective way to develop abdominal control while working your hip adductors, hip abductors, and quads. Working on one side at a time allows you to focus on multiple muscle groups.

ANNOTATION KEY
Black text indicates strengthening muscles
Gray text indicates stretching muscles
Italic text indicates tendons and ligaments
- - - - indicates deep muscles

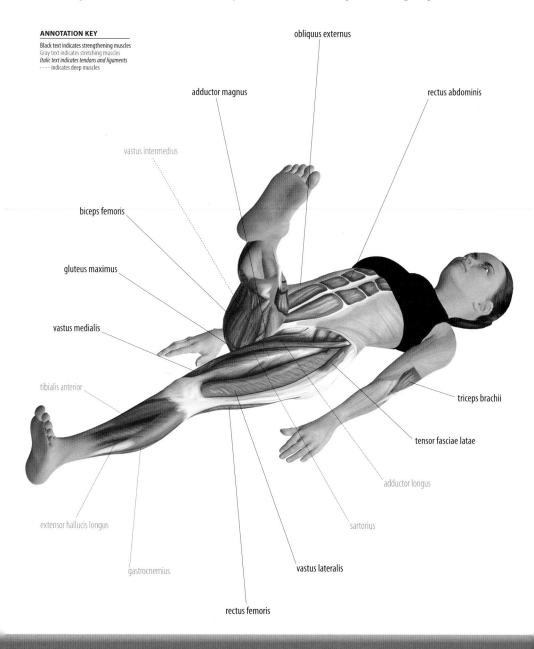

obliquus externus

adductor magnus

rectus abdominis

vastus intermedius

biceps femoris

gluteus maximus

vastus medialis

tibialis anterior

triceps brachii

tensor fasciae latae

adductor longus

extensor hallucis longus

sartorius

gastrocnemius

vastus lateralis

rectus femoris

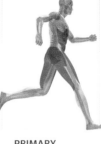

HOW TO DO IT

1 Lie flat on the floor with both arms and legs extended.

2 Bend your right knee toward your chest, and then straighten your leg up in the air. Anchor the rest of your body to the floor, straightening both knees and pressing your shoulders back and down.

3 Cross your raised leg up and over your body, aiming for your left shoulder.

Continue making a circle with the raised leg, returning to the center. Add emphasis to the motion by pausing at the top between repetitions.

4 Switch directions, and repeat. Lower your leg, and then repeat with the other leg. Complete full movement five to eight times.

PRIMARY TARGETS

- rectus abdominis
- obliquus externus
- rectus femoris
- biceps femoris
- triceps brachii
- gluteus maximus
- adductor magnus
- vastus lateralis
- vastus medialis
- tensor fasciae latae

BENEFITS

- Stabilizes pelvis
- Lengthens leg muscles
- Strengthens deep abdominal muscles

CAUTIONS

- Snapping hip syndrome—if this is an issue, reduce the size of the circles.

PERFECT YOUR FORM

- Keep your hips and torso stable while your legs are mobilized.
- Elongate your raised leg from your hip through your foot.
- Avoid making your leg circles too big to maintain stability.

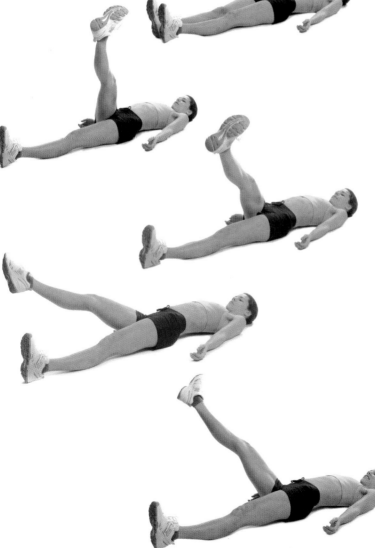

QUADRUPED LEG LIFT

BEGINNER

CONNECTING YOUR ARMS and legs with your core, while focusing on balancing and stability, is a key goal of the Quadruped Leg Lift. This exercise helps tone all the muscles along the body's central axis in one powerful, extending movement.

ANNOTATION KEY

Black text indicates strengthening muscles
Gray text indicates stretching muscles
Italic text indicates tendons and ligaments
- - - - indicates deep muscles

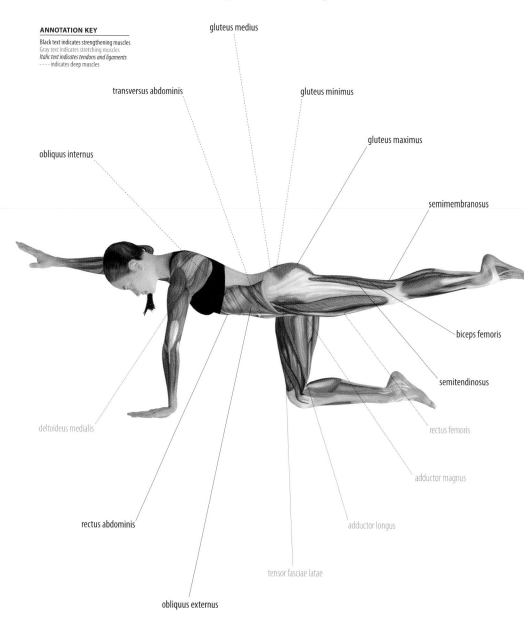

gluteus medius

transversus abdominis

gluteus minimus

gluteus maximus

obliquus internus

semimembranosus

biceps femoris

semitendinosus

deltoideus medialis

rectus femoris

adductor magnus

rectus abdominis

adductor longus

tensor fasciae latae

obliquus externus

HOW TO DO IT

1 Kneeling on all fours, connect with your abdominals by drawing your navel up toward your spine.

2 Slowly raise your right arm and extend your left leg, all while keeping your torso still. Extend your arm and leg until they are both parallel to the floor, creating one long line with your body. Do not allow your pelvis to bend or rotate.

3 Bring your arm and leg back into the starting position.

4 Repeat sequence on the other side, alternating sides six times.

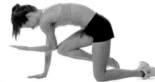

This variation will give your abs a greater challenge. Follow steps 1 and 2, and then draw your opposite knee and elbow inwards to touch. Repeat entire sequence on the other side.

PRIMARY TARGETS
- rectus abdominis
- transversus abdominis
- obliquus internus
- obliquus externus
- gluteus maximus
- gluteus minimus
- gluteus medius
- biceps femoris
- semitendinosus
- semimembranosus

BENEFITS
- Tones arms, legs, and abdominals

CAUTIONS
- Wrist pain
- Lower-back pain
- Knee pain
- Inability to stabilize the spine while moving limbs

PERFECT YOUR FORM
- Move slowly and steadily to decrease pelvic rotation.
- Engage your abs by drawing your navel toward your spine.

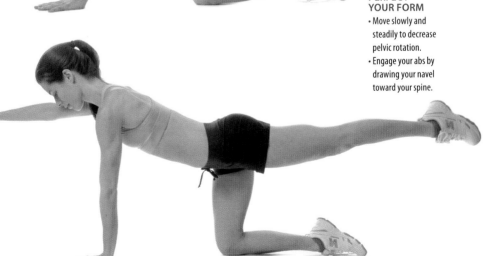

SWIMMING

BEGINNER

SWIMMING IS A FUN EXERCISE that calls on the same muscles that you use while swimming. Without stepping into a pool you will engage just about every muscle in your body. Use your exercise mat for stability, and aim for a long, full stretch in you arms and legs. As your head and shoulders come up off the mat, let your spine lengthen as well.

ANNOTATION KEY

Black text indicates strengthening muscles
Gray text indicates stretching muscles
Italic text indicates tendons and ligaments
- - - - indicates deep muscles

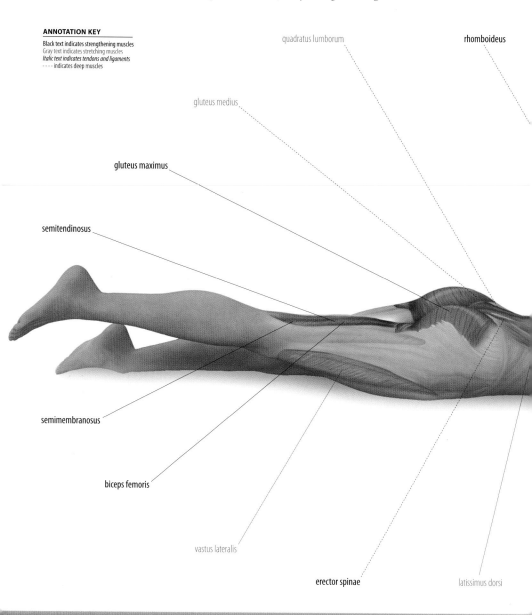

quadratus lumborum

rhomboideus

gluteus medius

gluteus maximus

semitendinosus

semimembranosus

biceps femoris

vastus lateralis

erector spinae

latissimus dorsi

HOW TO DO IT

1 Lie prone on the floor with your legs hip-width apart. Stretch your arms beside your ears on the floor. Engage your pelvic floor, and draw your navel into your spine.

2 Extend through your upper back as you lift your left arm and right leg simultaneously. Lift your head and shoulders off the floor.

3 Lower your arm and leg to the starting position, maintaining a stretch in your limbs throughout.

4 Extend your right arm and left leg off the floor, lengthening and lifting your head and shoulders.

5 Elongate your limbs as you return to the starting position. Repeat six to eight times.

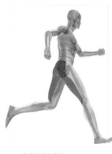

PRIMARY TARGETS
- gluteus maximus
- biceps femoris
- semitendinosus
- semimembranosus
- erector spinae
- rhomboideus

BENEFITS
- Strengthens hip and spine extensors
- Challenges stabilization of the spine against rotation

CAUTIONS
- Lower-back pain
- Extreme curvature of the upper spine
- Curvature of the lower spine

PERFECT YOUR FORM
- Extend your limbs as far as possible in opposite directions.
- Squeeze your glutes and draw your navel into your spine throughout.
- Keep your neck long and relaxed.
- Avoid allowing your shoulders to lift toward your ears.

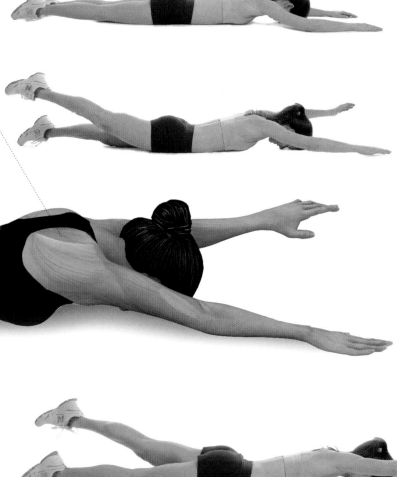

BICEPS CURL

BEGINNER

You use your arms mainly for balance when you run, but they can tire after a few miles. Include a few arm exercises in your work to strengthen your arms so that you can go the distance. The Biceps Curl is a basic movement that targets the biceps brachii—the two-headed muscle at the front of your upper arm.

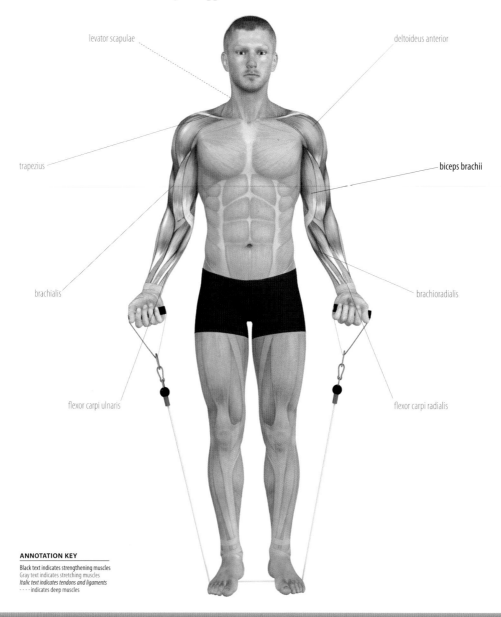

levator scapulae

deltoideus anterior

trapezius

biceps brachii

brachialis

brachioradialis

flexor carpi ulnaris

flexor carpi radialis

ANNOTATION KEY
Black text indicates strengthening muscles
Gray text indicates stretching muscles
Italic text indicates tendons and ligaments
- - - - indicates deep muscles

HOW TO DO IT

1 Stand upright with a resistance band beneath your feet. Your arms should be very slightly bent as you hold both handles of the resistance band in your hands, palms forward.

2 Curl the resistance band upward toward your shoulders.

3 Lower and repeat, completing three sets of 15.

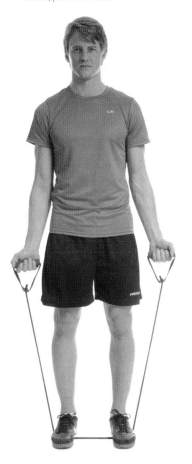
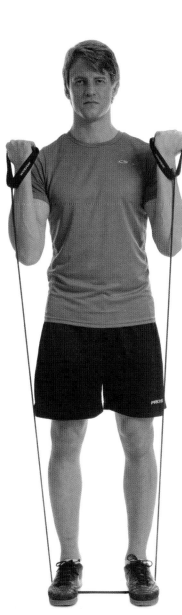

PRIMARY TARGETS
• biceps brachii

BENEFITS
• Strengthens and tones biceps

CAUTIONS
• Wrist or elbow pain

PERFECT YOUR FORM
• Keep your elbows at your sides.
• Don't rush through the exercise.

TRAINING YOUR SECONDARY MUSCLES

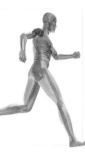

TRAINING YOUR SECONDARY MUSCLES

SWISS BALL SHOULDER PRESS

THE SWISS BALL SHOULDER PRESS targets your shoulders, especially the anterior deltoids. It also works your medial deltoids, along with your pectoral muscles and trapezius. Working on a ball adds a stability element, too, forcing you to keep your balance as you press upward.

PRIMARY TARGETS
- deltoideus anterior

BENEFITS
- Strengthens and tones front of shoulders

CAUTIONS
- Shoulder issues
- Rotator cuff injury

PERFECT YOUR FORM
- Pause at the top of the movement, and then lower to just above the start position, keeping tension on the muscles until the set is complete.
- Keep your elbows rigid without locking them at the top of the movement.
- Avoid tensing your neck.
- Avoid wiggling or squirming in an effort to press the weights upward.

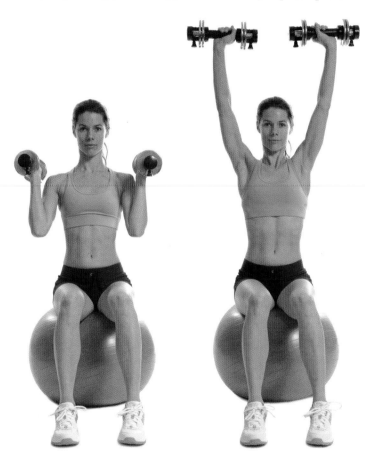

HOW TO DO IT

1 Sit on a Swiss ball in a well-balanced, neutral position, with your hips directly over the center of the ball, grasping a dumbbell in each hand. Hold one to each side of your shoulders with your elbows below wrists.

2 Press the dumbbells upward until your arms are fully extended overhead.

3 Lower to sides of shoulders and repeat for 10 to 15 repetitions.

TRICEPS EXTENSION

THE TRICEPS EXTENSION targets your triceps brachii muscle, the three-headed muscle at the back of your upper arm. To keep the focus on your triceps, keep your shoulders down and your elbow as close to your ear as possible, and avoid arching your back.

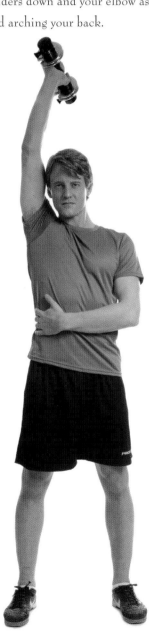

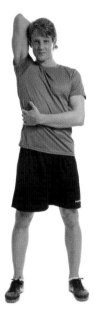

TRAINING YOUR SECONDARY MUSCLES

PRIMARY TARGETS
• triceps brachii

BENEFITS
• Strengthens and tones upper arms

CAUTIONS
• Shoulder issues
• Rotator cuff injury

PERFECT YOUR FORM
• Let the weight pull your arm back slightly to maintain full shoulder flexion.
• Keep your forearm in line with your ear throughout the exercise.
• Place your non-moving hand just under your ribs to stabilize your shoulder.
• Avoid dropping your elbow back or forward.

HOW TO DO IT

1 Stand with your legs and feet parallel and shoulder-width apart, grasping a dumbbell or hand weight in your right hand. Position the dumbbell over your head with your arm straight up or slightly back.

2 Lower the dumbbell behind your neck or shoulder while maintaining your upper arm's vertical position.

3 Extend your arm until straight. Repeat for 10 to 15 repetitions.

4 Return to starting position, and repeat on the opposite side.

LATERAL SHOULDER RAISE

BEGINNER

THE LATERAL SHOULDER RAISE is a weight-training exercise that will develop your medial deltoids. Your anterior deltoids, supraspinatus, trapezius, and serratus anterior assist in the movement, with the upper trapezius, levator scapulae, and wrist extensors acting as stabilizers to give your shoulders a full workout.

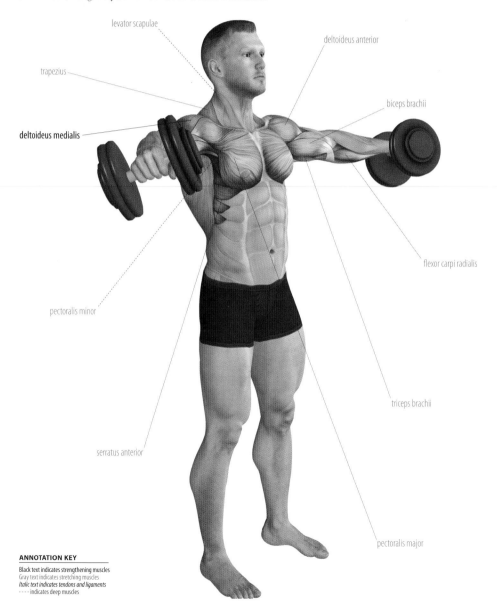

levator scapulae

deltoideus anterior

trapezius

biceps brachii

deltoideus medialis

flexor carpi radialis

pectoralis minor

triceps brachii

serratus anterior

pectoralis major

ANNOTATION KEY

Black text indicates strengthening muscles
Gray text indicates stretching muscles
Italic text indicates tendons and ligaments
- - - - indicates deep muscles

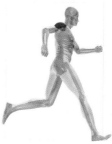

HOW TO DO IT

1 Holding a dumbbell in each hand, stand with your feet parallel and shoulder width apart, your knees slightly bent. Bend your elbow slightly and face your palms in toward your body.

2 Extend both arms out to the sides to shoulder height.

3 Slowly lower the dumbbells back to the starting position. Repeat, completing three sets of 10.

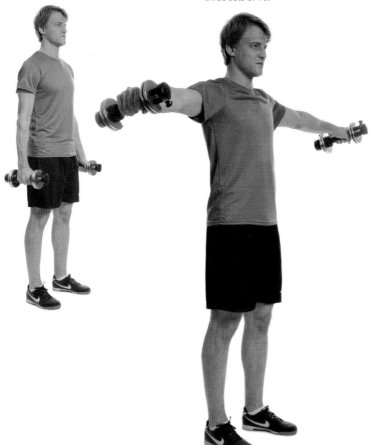

PRIMARY TARGETS
• deltoideus medialis

BENEFITS
• Strengthens medial deltoids
• Strengthens thoracic spine

CAUTIONS
• Acute rotator cuff injury

PERFECT YOUR FORM
• Keep your elbows in a fixed and slightly bent position throughout the movement.
• Position your elbows directly lateral to your shoulders at the top of the movement.
• Exhale as you lift the dumbbells, and inhale as you lower them.
• Keep your chest elevated.
• Keep your shoulders down.
• Avoid using momentum to lift the dumbbells.
• Avoid dropping your elbows lower than your wrists—this will make the front deltoids the primary movers instead of the lateral deltoids.

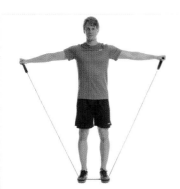

You can also perform this exercise with a resistance band. Secure it under both feet, and stand with your feet shoulder-width apart. With an end in each hand, extend both arms out to the sides to shoulder height. Slowly lower back to the starting position.

FRONTAL RAISE AND ROW

BEGINNER

THE FRONTAL RAISE AND ROW is a compound weight-training exercise. The raise portion of the exercise targets your anterior deltoids, while the row portion targets your posterior deltoids. Along the way, you also work the supporting muscles—the infraspinatus, teres minor, deltoideus medialis, trapezius, brachialis, brachioradialis, rhomboideus, and biceps brachii—giving your shoulders, upper arms, and upper back a workout, too.

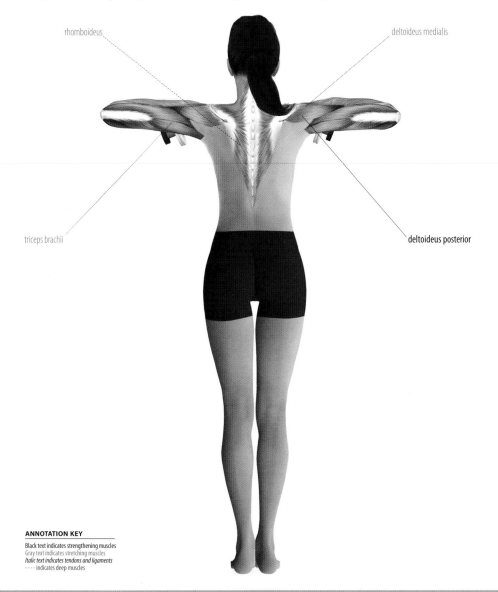

rhomboideus

deltoideus medialis

triceps brachii

deltoideus posterior

ANNOTATION KEY

Black text indicates strengthening muscles
Gray text indicates stretching muscles
Italic text indicates tendons and ligaments
- - - - indicates deep muscles

HOW TO DO IT

1 Holding a dumbbell or hand weight in each hand, stand with your legs and feet parallel and shoulder-width apart. Bend your knees very slightly and tuck your pelvis slightly forward, lift your chest, and press your shoulders downward and back.

2 Bring your arms up to a 90-degree angle from the front of the body.

3 Pull dumbbells to the front of your shoulders with your elbows leading out to sides.

4 Lower back to starting position, and repeat for two sets of 10.

PRIMARY TARGETS
- deltoideus anterior
- deltoideus medialis
- pectoralis major
- serratus anterior

BENEFITS
- Strengthens shoulders

CAUTIONS
- Shoulder issues
- Rotator cuff injury

PERFECT YOUR FORM
- Keep a slight bend in your elbow as you lift upward to avoid stress on the joints.

- Avoid raising your elbows or the weight higher than your shoulders.

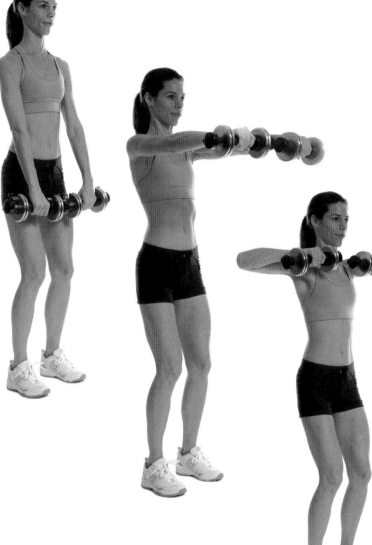

PUSH-UP

BEGINNER

THE CLASSIC PUSH-UP is found in just about every workout regimen, from high school physical education to military basic training. Push-Ups target the pectoral muscles, triceps, and anterior deltoids, with secondary benefits to your posterior and medial deltoids, serratus anterior, coracobrachialis, and your entire midsection.

ANNOTATION KEY
Black text indicates strengthening muscles
Gray text indicates stretching muscles
Italic text indicates tendons and ligaments
- - - - indicates deep muscles

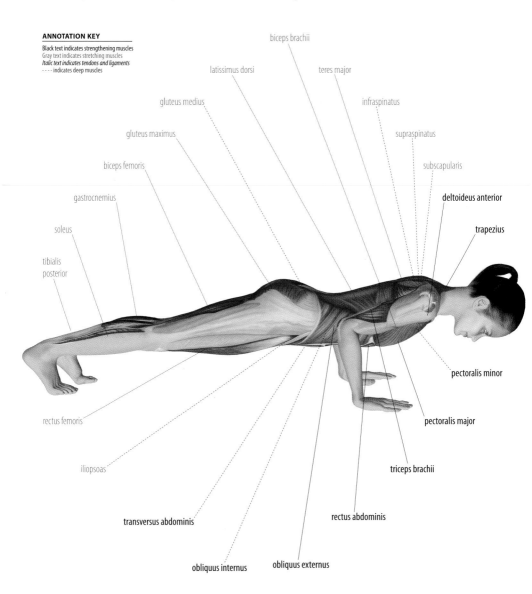

biceps brachii

latissimus dorsi

teres major

gluteus medius

infraspinatus

gluteus maximus

supraspinatus

biceps femoris

subscapularis

gastrocnemius

deltoideus anterior

soleus

trapezius

tibialis posterior

pectoralis minor

rectus femoris

pectoralis major

iliopsoas

triceps brachii

transversus abdominis

rectus abdominis

obliquus internus

obliquus externus

HOW TO DO IT

1 From a standing position, bend forward and walk your hands out until they are directly beneath your shoulders in a high plank position.

2 Inhale, and set your body by drawing your abdominals to your spine. Squeeze your buttocks and legs together and stretch out of your heels, bringing your body into a straight line.

3 Exhale and inhale as you bend your elbows and lower your body toward the floor.

4 Push upward to return to plank position. Keep your elbows close to your body. Repeat eight times.

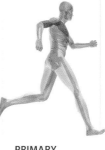

PRIMARY TARGETS
- triceps brachii
- pectoralis major
- pectoralis minor
- coracobrachialis
- deltoideus anterior
- rectus abdominis
- transversus abdominis
- obliquus externus
- obliquus internus
- trapezius

BENEFITS
- Strengthens the core stabilizers, shoulders, back, glutes, and pectoral muscles

CAUTIONS
- Shoulder issues
- Wrist pain
- Lower-back pain

PERFECT YOUR FORM
- Relax your neck, keeping it long as you perform the upward movement.
- Squeeze your glutes as you scoop in your abdominals for stability.
- Avoid allowing your shoulders to lift towards your ears.

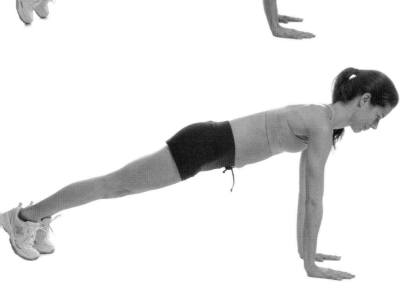

BASIC CRUNCH

BEGINNER

THE BASIC CRUNCH is one of the go-to exercises for toning your abdominals. Crunches are highly effective at isolating the rectus abdominis. This paired muscle, which runs vertically on each side of the anterior wall of the abdomen, is an important postural muscle, as well as one of respiration, allowing you to forcefully exhale, as when running. To ease any lumbar strain, while performing crunches try to keep your lower back on the floor throughout the entire set of repetitions.

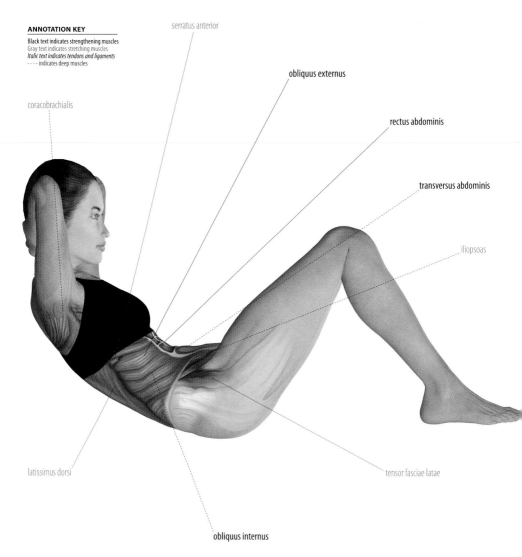

ANNOTATION KEY

Black text indicates strengthening muscles
Gray text indicates stretching muscles
Italic text indicates tendons and ligaments
- - - - indicates deep muscles

serratus anterior

obliquus externus

coracobrachialis

rectus abdominis

transversus abdominis

iliopsoas

latissimus dorsi

tensor fasciae latae

obliquus internus

HOW TO DO IT

1 Lie on your back with your knees bent, and clasp your hands behind your head.

2 Keeping your elbows wide, engage your abdominals, and lift your upper torso to achieve a crunching movement.

3 Slowly return to the starting position. Repeat 15 times for two sets.

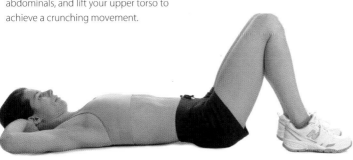

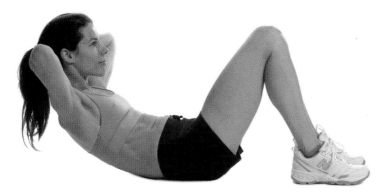

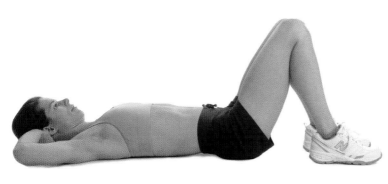

PRIMARY TARGETS
- rectus abdominis
- obliquus internus
- obliquus externus
- transversus abdominis

BENEFITS
- Strengthens the torso
- Improves pelvic and core stability

CAUTIONS
- Back pain
- Neck pain

PERFECT YOUR FORM
- Use your shoulders and abdominals to initiate the movement.
- Keep your pelvis in neutral position during the crunch.
- Slightly tuck your chin, directing your gaze toward your inner thighs.
- Avoid pulling from the neck.
- Avoid tilting your hips towards the floor.

CROSSOVER CRUNCH

INTERMEDIATE

THE CROSSOVER CRUNCH, which targets the oblique muscles, not only helps define your waist, but also strengthens and stabilizes your core so that you can run with the best form possible. Adding this exercise to your regimen will leave you with abdominals that are more toned and a back that has greater rotational flexibility.

ANNOTATION KEY

Black text indicates strengthening muscles
Gray text indicates stretching muscles
Italic text indicates tendons and ligaments
- - - - indicates deep muscles

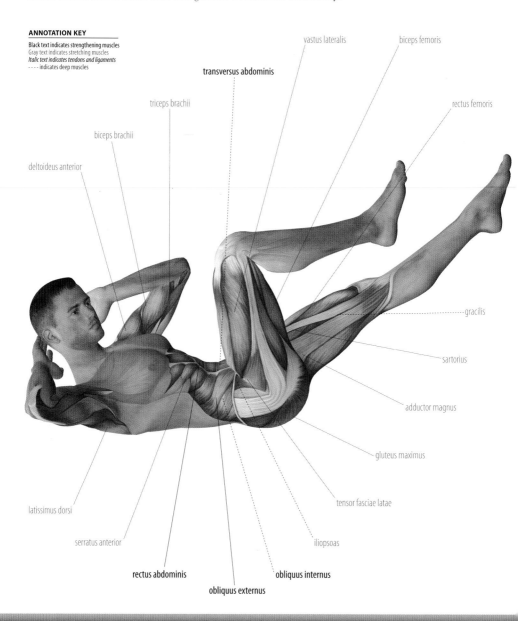

vastus lateralis

biceps femoris

transversus abdominis

triceps brachii

rectus femoris

biceps brachii

deltoideus anterior

gracilis

sartorius

adductor magnus

gluteus maximus

tensor fasciae latae

latissimus dorsi

iliopsoas

serratus anterior

rectus abdominis

obliquus internus

obliquus externus

HOW TO DO IT

1 Lie on your back with your hands behind your head. Lift your legs into a tabletop position, so that your thighs and calves form a 90-degree angle with your thighs parallel to the floor.

2 Roll up with your torso, reaching your right elbow to your left knee and extending your right leg in front of you.

Imagine pulling your shoulder blades off the floor and twisting from your ribs and oblique muscles.

3 Alternate extending your right and left legs. Repeat sequence six times.

PRIMARY TARGETS
- rectus abdominis
- transversus abdominis
- obliquus externus
- obliquus internus

BENEFITS
- Stabilizes core
- Strengthens abdominals

CAUTIONS
- Neck issues
- Lower-back pain

PERFECT YOUR FORM
- Elongate your neck.
- Lift your chin away from your chest.
- Keep both hips stable on the floor.
- Avoid pulling with your hands.
- Avoid arching your back.
- Avoid moving the active elbow faster than your shoulder.

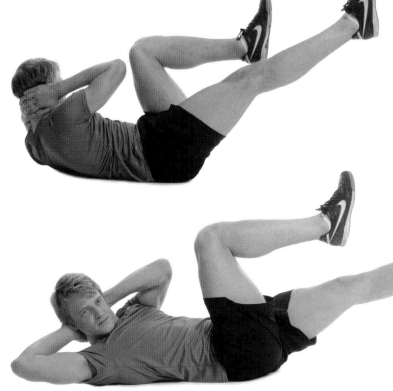

TRAINING YOUR SECONDARY MUSCLES

ABDOMINAL KICK

INTERMEDIATE

The Abdominal Kick stabilizes your entire core and strengthens your abdominal muscles, especially your transversus abdominis, or lower abs. This exercise trains you to move from your center, using your abdominal muscles to initiate movement and to support and stabilize your trunk as your arms and legs are in motion. It can also help improve your overall coordination.

ANNOTATION KEY

Black text indicates strengthening muscles
Gray text indicates stretching muscles
Italic text indicates tendons and ligaments
- - - - indicates deep muscles

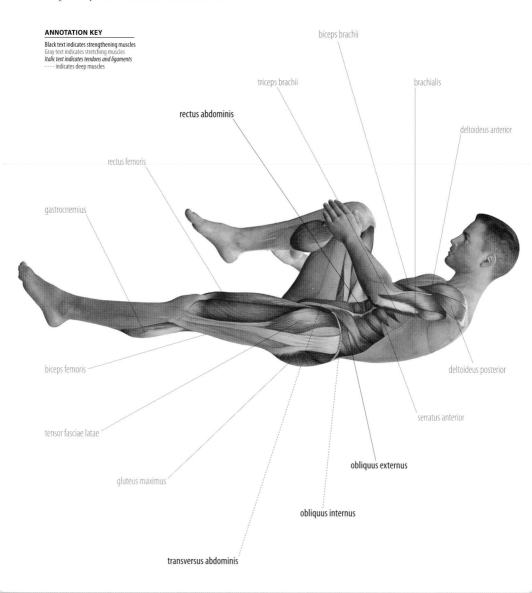

biceps brachii

triceps brachii

brachialis

rectus abdominis

deltoideus anterior

rectus femoris

gastrocnemius

biceps femoris

deltoideus posterior

tensor fasciae latae

serratus anterior

obliquus externus

gluteus maximus

obliquus internus

transversus abdominis

HOW TO DO IT

1 Lie on your back with your legs extended. Pull your right knee toward your chest and straighten your left leg, raising it 45 degrees from the floor.

2 Place your right hand on your right ankle and your left hand on your right knee to maintain proper leg alignment.

3 Switch your legs two times, switching your hand placement simultaneously.

4 Switch your legs two more times, keeping your hands in their proper placement. Repeat four to six times.

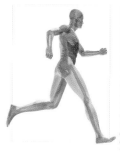

PRIMARY TARGETS
• rectus abdominis
• transversus abdominis
• obliquus externus
• obliquus internus

BENEFITS
• Stabilizes core while extremities are in motion
• Strengthens abdominals

CAUTIONS
• Neck issues
• Lower-back pain

PERFECT YOUR FORM
• Place your outside hand on the ankle of your bent leg and your inside hand on your bent knee.
• Lift your chest.
• Avoid allowing your lower back to rise off the floor; use your abdominals to stabilize your core while switching legs.

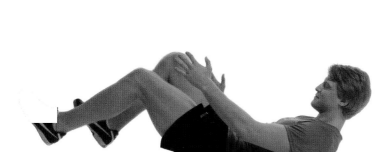

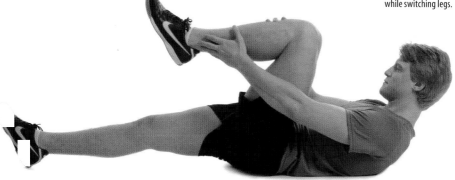

STANDING KNEE CRUNCH

INTERMEDIATE

THE STANDING KNEE CRUNCH has all the benefits of a Basic Crunch—strengthening your abdominals—while also challenging your coordination and sense of balance.

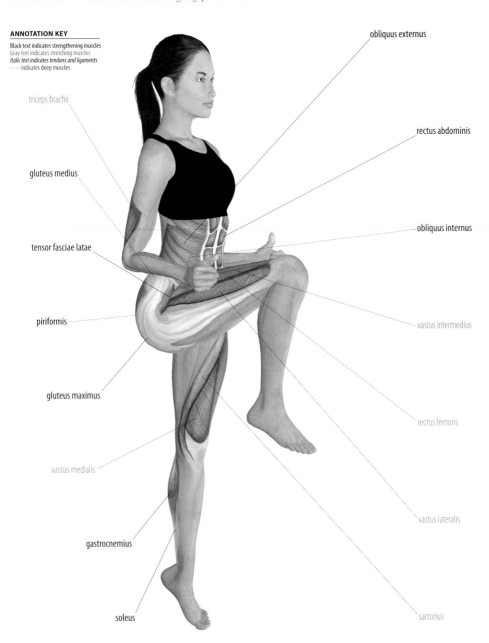

ANNOTATION KEY

Black text indicates strengthening muscles
Gray text indicates stretching muscles
Italic text indicates tendons and ligaments
- - - - indicates deep muscles

obliquus externus

triceps brachii

rectus abdominis

gluteus medius

obliquus internus

tensor fasciae latae

vastus intermedius

piriformis

gluteus maximus

rectus femoris

vastus medialis

vastus lateralis

gastrocnemius

soleus

sartorius

HOW TO DO IT

1 Stand tall with your left leg in front of the right, and extend your hands toward the ceiling, your arms straight.

2 Shift your weight onto your left foot, and raise your right knee to the height of your hips. To create the crunch, simultaneously lift up on the toes of your left leg, while pulling your elbows down by your sides, your hands making fists.

3 Pause at the top of the movement, and then return to the starting position. Repeat the sequence with your right leg as the standing leg. Repeat 10 times on each leg.

PRIMARY TARGETS
- rectus abdominis
- obliquus internus
- obliquus externus
- transversus abdominis
- gluteus maximus
- gluteus medius
- tensor fasciae latae
- piriformis
- iliopsoas
- gastrocnemius
- soleus

BENEFITS
- Strengthens core
- Strengthens calves and gluteal muscles
- Improves balance

CAUTIONS
- Knee pain

PERFECT YOUR FORM
- Keep your standing leg straight as you rise up on your toes.
- Relax your shoulders as you pull your arms down for the crunch.
- Flex the toes of your raised leg.
- Avoid tilting forward as you switch legs.

ILIOTIBIAL BAND RELEASE

INTERMEDIATE

A TIGHT OR INFLAMED ILIOTIBIAL BAND is a bane to even the most experienced runners, sidelining them for weeks or even longer. Strengthening the hip muscles that support the iliotibial band can prevent injury, and releasing it through massage can relieve any tension. In this exercise, you use a dense foam roller to administer a self-massage from high hip to knee, down the entire length of the band.

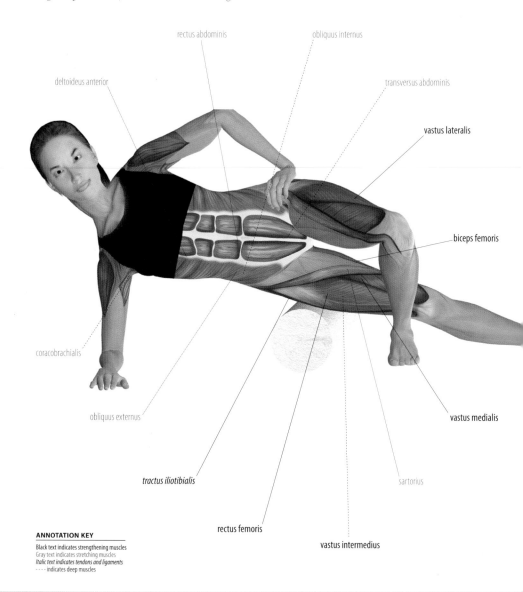

rectus abdominis

obliquus internus

deltoideus anterior

transversus abdominis

vastus lateralis

biceps femoris

coracobrachialis

obliquus externus

vastus medialis

tractus iliotibialis

sartorius

rectus femoris

vastus intermedius

ANNOTATION KEY

Black text indicates strengthening muscles
Gray text indicates stretching muscles
Italic text indicates tendons and ligaments
- - - - indicates deep muscles

HOW TO DO IT

1 Lie on your right side, with a foam roller placed under the middle of your thigh. Support your torso with your right forearm on the floor.

2 Bend your left leg and cross it in front of your right, so that your knee is pointed upward. Place your left foot flat on the floor.

3 Pulling with your shoulder and pushing with your supporting leg, roll back and forth along the side of your thigh. Adjust the placement of your arm as you make your motion bigger.

4 Repeat 15 times on each side.

PRIMARY TARGETS
- tractus iliotibialis
- rectus femoris
- vastus medialis
- vastus intermedius
- vastus lateralis
- biceps femoris
- infraspinatus
- supraspinatus
- teres minor
- subscapularis

BENEFITS
- Releases the iliotibial band
- Strengthens the scapular stabilizers and lateral trunk muscles

CAUTIONS
- Shoulder pain
- Back pain

PERFECT YOUR FORM
- Relax your shoulders.
- Press your hands and forearms firmly into the floor.
- Avoid allowing your shoulders to lift toward your ears.

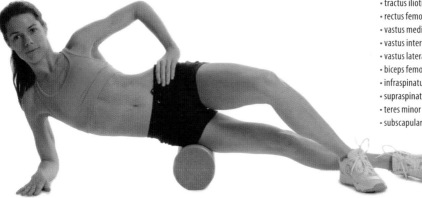

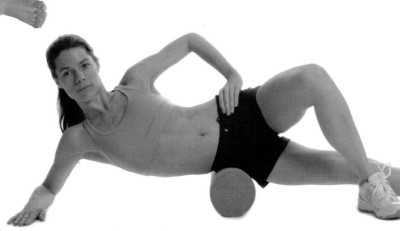

SWISS BALL PUSH-UP

INTERMEDIATE

ADD AN EXTRA CHALLENGE to the basic Push-Up by performing it with your feet propped on a Swiss ball. This demanding exercise works your chest, shoulders, triceps, and core.

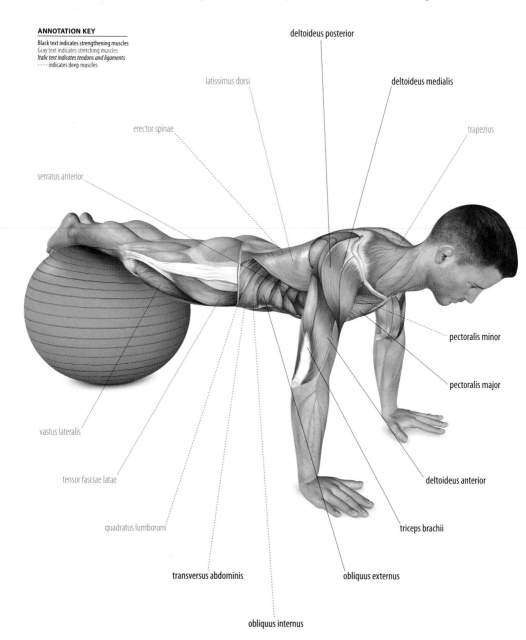

ANNOTATION KEY

Black text indicates strengthening muscles
Gray text indicates stretching muscles
Italic text indicates tendons and ligaments
---- indicates deep muscles

deltoideus posterior

latissimus dorsi

deltoideus medialis

erector spinae

trapezius

serratus anterior

pectoralis minor

pectoralis major

vastus lateralis

tensor fasciae latae

deltoideus anterior

triceps brachii

quadratus lumborum

transversus abdominis

obliquus externus

obliquus internus

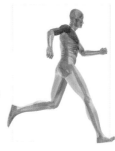

HOW TO DO IT

1 Place your toes on top of a Swiss ball, and walk your arms out until your legs are fully extended and your body forms a straight line from shoulders to feet, your hands shoulder-width apart.

2 Lower your torso until your chest almost touches the floor.

3 Press your upper body back up to the starting position and squeeze your chest muscles. Pause at the contracted position, and repeat the flexing and extending at your elbows for three sets of 10 repetitions.

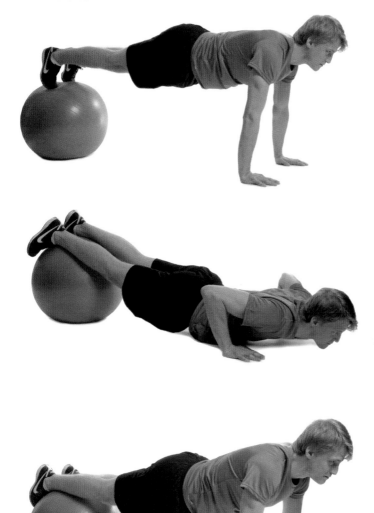

PRIMARY TARGETS
- pectoralis major
- pectoralis minor
- deltoideus posterior
- deltoideus anterior
- deltoideus medialis
- triceps brachii
- transversus abdominis
- obliquus externus
- obliquus internus

BENEFITS
- Strengthens shoulders
- Stabilizes core
- Strengthens abdominals

CAUTIONS
- Wrist pain
- Lower-back pain
- Shoulder instability

PERFECT YOUR FORM
- Form a straight plane from neck to ankles.
- Inhale as you lower your torso, and exhale as you press back up.
- Avoid arching your back during the exercise.
- Avoid rotating your hips.
- Avoid locking your elbows.

SWISS BALL WALKOUT

INTERMEDIATE

THE SWISS BALL WALKOUT challenges your core, while working your chest, back, and arm muscles. The unstable surface of the ball demands that you move with steadiness and control, which will enhance your coordination and sense of balance.

ANNOTATION KEY
Black text indicates strengthening muscles
Gray text indicates stretching muscles
Italic text indicates tendons and ligaments
- - - - indicates deep muscles

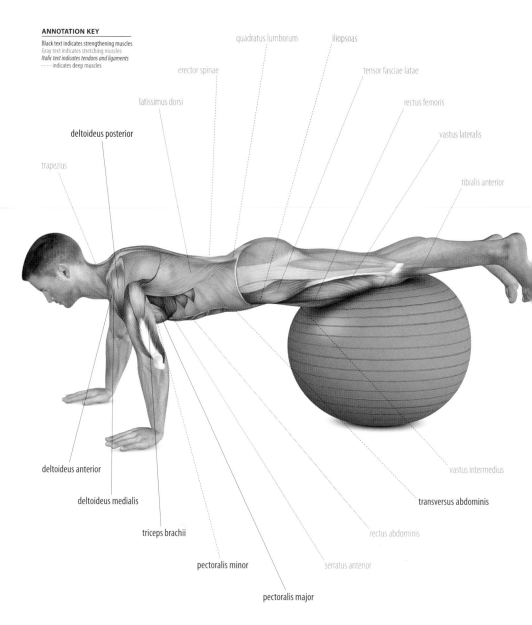

quadratus lumborum

iliopsoas

erector spinae

tensor fasciae latae

latissimus dorsi

rectus femoris

deltoideus posterior

vastus lateralis

trapezius

tibialis anterior

deltoideus anterior

vastus intermedius

deltoideus medialis

transversus abdominis

triceps brachii

rectus abdominis

pectoralis minor

serratus anterior

pectoralis major

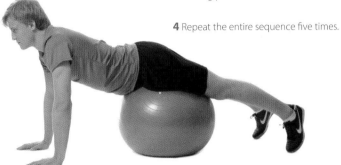

HOW TO DO IT

1 Lie prone on a Swiss ball, with your hips positioned directly over the center of the ball as you support your weight on your arms. Place your hands directly below your shoulders.

2 Lift, reach, and place your left hand forward, rolling the ball underneath you until it reaches your feet.

3 Hold for 5 seconds, and then walk your hands backward, rolling the ball back underneath you until you reach the starting position.

4 Repeat the entire sequence five times.

TRAINING YOUR SECONDARY MUSCLES

PRIMARY TARGETS
- deltoideus anterior
- deltoideus medialis
- deltoideus posterior
- transversus abdominis
- triceps brachii
- pectoralis major
- pectoralis minor

BENEFITS
- Strengthens shoulders
- Stabilizes core
- Strengthens abdominals

CAUTIONS
- Wrist pain
- Lower-back pain
- Shoulder instability

PERFECT YOUR FORM
- Form a straight plane from neck to ankles.
- Activate your abdominals as you straighten your back.
- Avoid arching your back during the exercise.
- Avoid allowing your hips to rotate.
- Avoid locking your elbows.
- Don't reach too far forward—start with a short reach position and progressively increase the length as you gain stability.

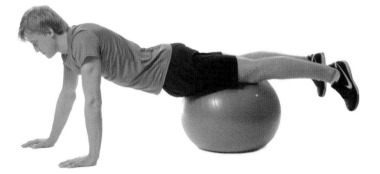

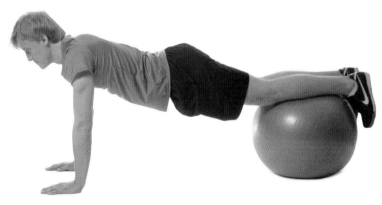

SWISS BALL EXTENSION

ADVANCED

BACK EXTENSIONS are excellent exercises to strengthen your lower back, working the erector spinae muscles on either side of your spine. Performing the Swiss Ball Extension adds both an element of support and a greater challenge because you must fully engage your core muscles to stabilize your entire body.

ANNOTATION KEY
Black text indicates strengthening muscles
Gray text indicates stretching muscles
Italic text indicates tendons and ligaments
- - - - indicates deep muscles

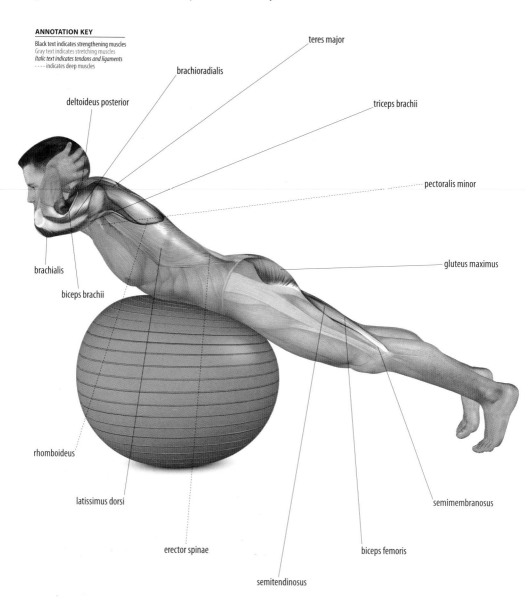

teres major

brachioradialis

deltoideus posterior

triceps brachii

pectoralis minor

brachialis

biceps brachii

gluteus maximus

rhomboideus

latissimus dorsi

semimembranosus

erector spinae

biceps femoris

semitendinosus

HOW TO DO IT

1 Lie prone over a Swiss ball, with your upper chest and head hanging off the edge of the ball.

2 Firmly plant your feet to stabilize yourself over the ball, and place your hands on either side of your head.

3 With arms bent and elbows out, raise your upper body off the ball.

4 Slowly and carefully lower your body to the starting position. Repeat 10 times.

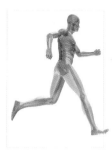

PRIMARY TARGETS
- erector spinae
- gluteus maximus
- biceps femoris
- semitendinosus
- semimembranosus
- adductor magnus
- latissimus dorsi
- teres major
- triceps brachii
- deltoideus posterior
- brachialis
- brachioradialis
- biceps brachii
- trapezius
- pectoralis minor
- rhomboideus
- multifidus spinae

BENEFITS
- Stabilizes core
- Strengthens back extensor muscles and abdominals

CAUTIONS
- Neck issues
- Lower-back pain

PERFECT YOUR FORM
- Engage your glutes and thighs throughout the exercise.
- Keep your head in neutral position.
- Maintain a wide base for extra balance.

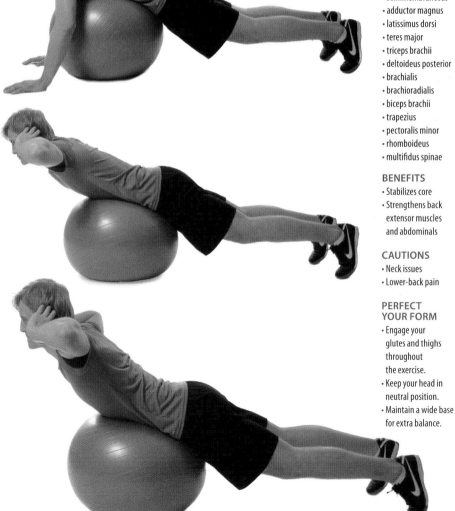

BACKWARD BALL STRETCH

ADVANCED

ANOTHER EXERCISE that enhances your coordination, the Backward Ball Stretch is both an abdominal and back stretch and a core-strengthening exercise. You must fully engage your core, using steady, controlled movement to stretch back over the unstable ball.

ANNOTATION KEY

Black text indicates strengthening muscles
Gray text indicates stretching muscles
Italic text indicates tendons and ligaments
- - - - indicates deep muscles

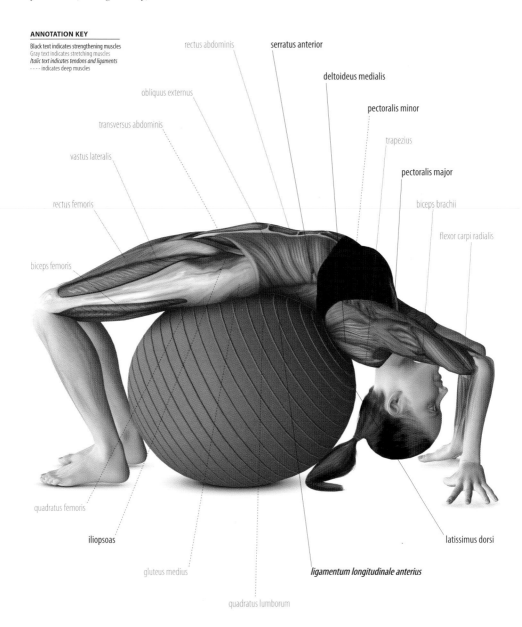

rectus abdominis

serratus anterior

deltoideus medialis

pectoralis minor

trapezius

pectoralis major

biceps brachii

flexor carpi radialis

obliquus externus

transversus abdominis

vastus lateralis

rectus femoris

biceps femoris

quadratus femoris

iliopsoas

gluteus medius

quadratus lumborum

ligamentum longitudinale anterius

latissimus dorsi

HOW TO DO IT

1 Sit on a Swiss ball in a well-balanced, neutral position, with your hips directly over the center of the ball.

2 While maintaining good balance, begin to extend your arms behind you.

3 Walk your feet forward, allowing the ball to roll up your spine.

4 As your hands touch the floor, extend your legs as far forward as you comfortably can. Hold this position for 10 seconds.

5 To deepen the stretch, extend your arms and walk your legs and hands closer to the ball. Hold this position for 10 seconds.

6 To release the stretch, bend your knees, drop your hips to the floor, lift your head off the ball, and then walk back to the starting position.

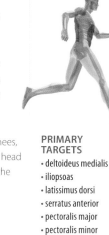

PRIMARY TARGETS
- deltoideus medialis
- iliopsoas
- latissimus dorsi
- serratus anterior
- pectoralis major
- pectoralis minor
- ligamentum longitudinale anterius

BENEFITS
- Stretches thoracic spine
- Increases spinal extension
- Stretches abdominals and large back muscles

CAUTIONS
- Lower-back pain
- Balancing difficulty

PERFECT YOUR FORM
- Maintain good balance throughout the stretch.
- Move slowly and in a controlled manner.
- Keep your head on the ball until you have dropped your knees all the way down as you release from the stretch.
- Avoid allowing the ball to shift to the side.
- Avoid holding the extended position for too long, or until you feel dizzy.

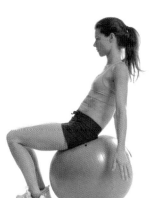

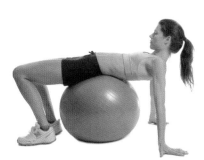

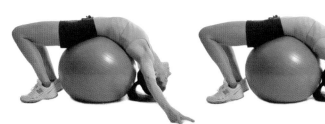

FRONT PLANK EXTENSION

ADVANCED

PACKING A POWERFUL PUNCH, the Front Plank Extension targets your leg, abdominal, shoulder, and arm muscles. This exercise calls for you to maintain a stable position while achieving full-body extension and flexion.

ANNOTATION KEY
Black text indicates strengthening muscles
Gray text indicates stretching muscles
Italic text indicates tendons and ligaments
- - - - indicates deep muscles

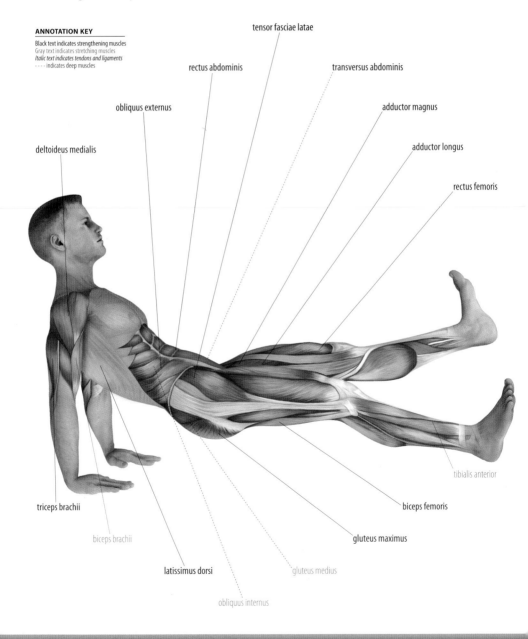

tensor fasciae latae

rectus abdominis

transversus abdominis

obliquus externus

adductor magnus

deltoideus medialis

adductor longus

rectus femoris

tibialis anterior

triceps brachii

biceps femoris

biceps brachii

gluteus maximus

latissimus dorsi

gluteus medius

obliquus internus

HOW TO DO IT

1 Sit with your legs parallel and extended out in front of you. Place your hands behind you with your fingers pointed toward your hips.

2 Press up through your arms and lift your chest up, squeezing your glutes and lifting your hips while pressing your heels into the floor. Continue lifting your pelvis until your body forms a long line from your shoulders to your feet.

3 Without allowing your pelvis to drop, keep your left leg straight, and raise it as high as you comfortably can.

4 Slowly lower it to the floor, and switch to the right leg. Repeat four to six times on each side.

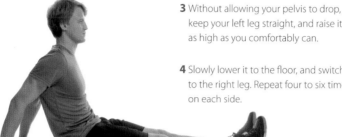

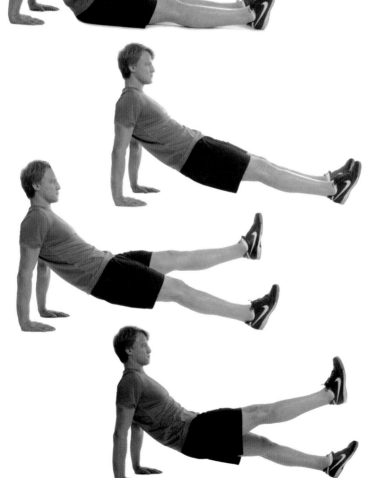

PRIMARY TARGETS

- gluteus maximus
- biceps femoris
- deltoideus
- rectus femoris
- adductor magnus
- tensor fasciae latae
- rectus abdominis
- transversus abdominis
- adductor longus
- obliquus externus
- latissimus dorsi
- triceps brachii

BENEFITS

- Strengthens core muscles and deep stabilizing muscles

CAUTIONS

- Wrist pain
- Knee pain
- Shoulder injury
- Shooting pains down leg

PERFECT YOUR FORM

- Elevate your pelvis throughout the exercise.
- Avoid allowing your shoulders to sink into their sockets.
- If your legs do not feel strong enough to support your body, slightly bend your knees.

ROLLER BRIDGE WITH LEG LIFT

ADVANCED

THE ROLLER BRIDGE LEG LIFT targets your abdominals, glutes, and hamstrings, while improving your pelvis stability. Like a Swiss ball, the foam roller provides an element of instability, which really challenges your sense of balance and coordination.

ANNOTATION KEY
Black text indicates strengthening muscles
Gray text indicates stretching muscles
Italic text indicates tendons and ligaments
- - - - indicates deep muscles

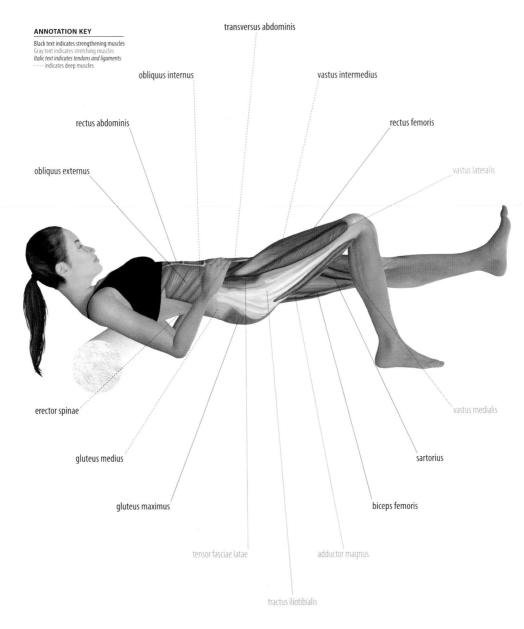

transversus abdominis

obliquus internus

vastus intermedius

rectus abdominis

rectus femoris

obliquus externus

vastus lateralis

erector spinae

vastus medialis

gluteus medius

sartorius

gluteus maximus

biceps femoris

tensor fasciae latae

adductor magnus

tractus iliotibialis

HOW TO DO IT

1 Lie on your back, with a foam roller under your shoulders. Your buttocks should be on the floor, with your knees bent and feet flat on the floor.

2 Press into the floor with your feet and bridge upward, lifting your hips toward the ceiling until they are flat and parallel to the floor.

3 Extend your right leg.

4 Raise your right leg up to the height of your knees. Keeping your leg straight and the roller still, raise and lower your hips.

5 Return to step 2, and then repeat step 3 and step 4 with your left leg.

6 Repeat 15 times on each leg.

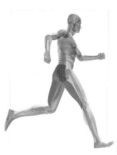

PRIMARY TARGETS
- rectus abdominis
- transversus abdominis
- obliquus internus
- obliquus externus
- gluteus maximus
- gluteus medius
- vastus intermedius
- rectus femoris
- sartorius
- biceps femoris
- erector spinae

BENEFITS
- Improves pelvic stabilization
- Strengthens gluteal muscles
- Strengthens hamstrings

CAUTIONS
- Hamstring injury
- Lower-back pain
- Ankle pain

PERFECT YOUR FORM
- Keep your extended leg straight.
- Avoid allowing your hips and lower back to drop during the movement.
- Avoid arching your back.

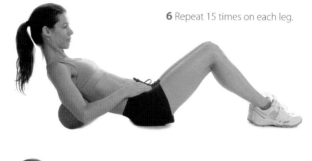

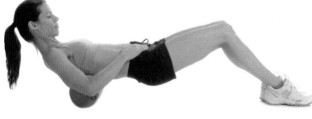

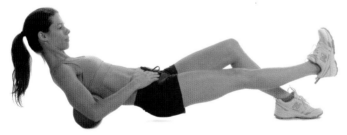

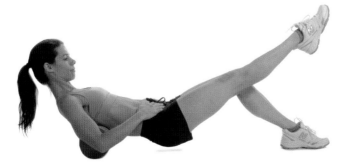

THREE-LEGGED DOG

ADVANCED

THIS EXERCISE IS A VARIATION of the traditional Downward-Facing Dog posture of yoga, which calls for you to balance on all four limbs to strengthen your arm and leg muscles and create space in your torso for better organ function. Three-Legged Dog adds a further challenge by adding a backward leg extension to an asymmetrical balance.

ANNOTATION KEY

Black text indicates strengthening muscles
Gray text indicates stretching muscles
Italic text indicates tendons and ligaments
- - - - indicates deep muscles

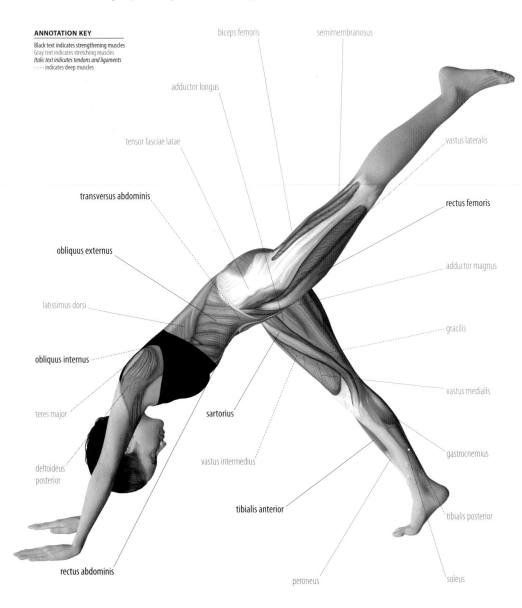

biceps femoris

semimembranosus

adductor longus

tensor fasciae latae

vastus lateralis

transversus abdominis

rectus femoris

obliquus externus

adductor magnus

latissimus dorsi

gracilis

obliquus internus

vastus medialis

teres major

sartorius

deltoideus posterior

vastus intermedius

gastrocnemius

tibialis anterior

tibialis posterior

rectus abdominis

peroneus

soleus

HOW TO DO IT

1 Start in plank position, with your shoulders directly over your hands, your torso straight, and your weight distributed evenly between your arms and legs.

2 Draw your left knee into your chest, flexing your foot while rocking your body forward over your hands. You should come up on the toes of your right foot.

3 Extend your left knee backward, rocking the body back, and shifting your weight onto your heel. With your head in between your hands, straighten your right leg and lift it towards the ceiling. Repeat 10 times on each leg.

PRIMARY TARGETS
- rectus abdominis
- transversus abdominis
- sartorius
- obliquus externus
- obliquus internus
- rectus femoris
- tibialis anterior

BENEFITS
- Stabilizes core
- Stabilizes shoulders
- Stretches calves and hamstrings

CAUTIONS
- Sharp lower-back pain
- Wrist pain
- Ankle pain

PERFECT YOUR FORM
- Align your shoulders over your hands.
- Flex your toes inward during the movement.
- Avoid bending the knee of the supporting leg.

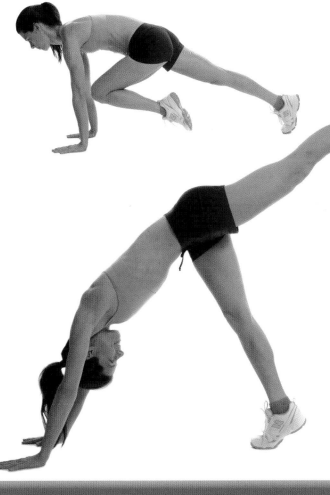

TRAINING YOUR SECONDARY MUSCLES

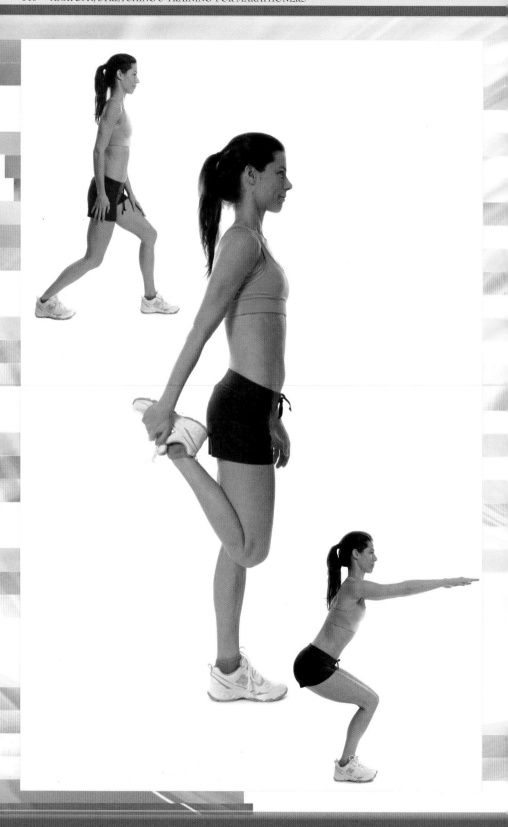

TRAINING WORKOUTS

Once you have gone through the stretching and strengthening exercises in this book and practiced executing them properly, your next step is to put these moves together. The following sequences are just samples of the many ways that you can combine these exercises to create marathon training warm-ups and cool-downs, as well as targeted or all-over strengthening workouts. They provide flexible frameworks that you can adapt to accommodate your specific fitness level or area of concern—if you want to avoid a certain exercise in any one of them, simply substitute another that has a similar benefit. Try the workouts featured here, adding them to your training schedule workout days, and then flip through the exercises and create your own stretching routines and strengthening and stability workouts to suit your individual goals.

BEGINNER STRETCHING ROUTINE

Perform this series of stretches before you run and as a cool-down post-run.

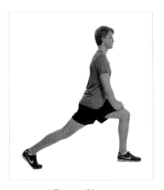

1 Forward Lunge
page 34

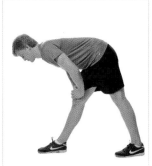

2 Straight-Leg Lunge
page 36

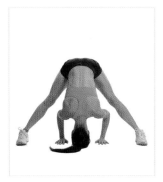

3 Wide-Legged Forward Bend
page 38

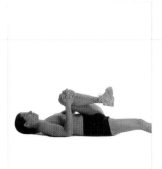

4 Knee-to-Chest Hug
page 44

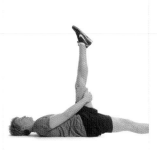

5 Unilateral Leg Raise
page 60

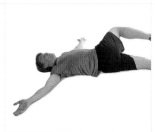

6 Spinal Rotation Stretch
page 62

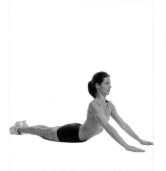

7 Cobra Stretch
page 58

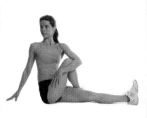

8 Hip/Iliotibial Band Stretch
page 64

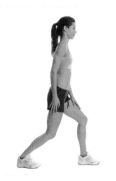

9 Calf Stretch
page 54

INTERMEDIATE STRETCHING ROUTINE

Try these stretches both pre- and post-run, adding new ones as your training progresses.

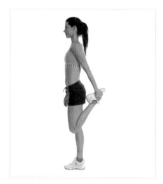

1 Standing Quads Stretch
page 30

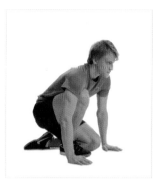

2 Sprinter's Stretch
page 32

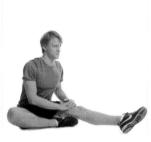

3 Unilateral Seated
Forward Bend
page 42

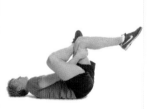

4 Supine Figure 4
page 46

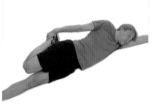

5 Side-Lying Knee Bend
page 48

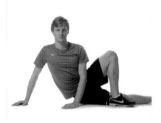

6 Side-Lying Rib Stretch
page 50

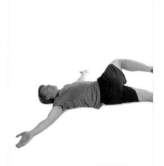

7 Spinal Rotation Stretch
page 62

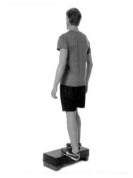

8 Heel-Drop/Toe-Up Stretch
page 52

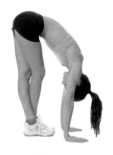

9 Iliotibial Band Stretch
page 64

ADVANCED STRETCHING ROUTINE

This balanced series of stretches works all your primary running muscles.

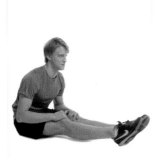

1 Bilateral Seated
Forward Bend
page 40

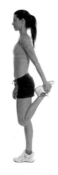

2 Standing Quads Stretch
page 30

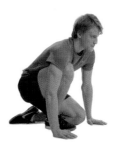

3 Sprinter's Stretch
page 32

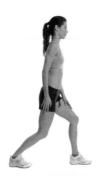

4 Calf Stretch
page 54

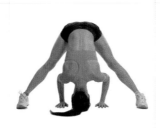

5 Wide-Legged Forward Bend
page 38

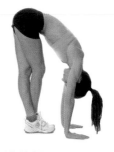

6 Iliotibial Band Stretch
page 64

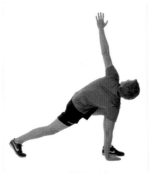

7 Forward Lunge with Twist
page 66

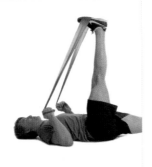

8 Tendon Stretch
page 70

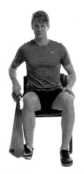

9 Ankle Stretches
page 71

BEGINNER STRENGTHENING WORKOUT

This series of exercises will help you begin building strength in the key running muscles.

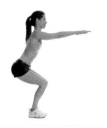

1 Knee Squat
page 80

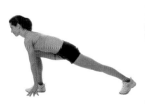

2 Yoga Lunge
page 86

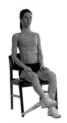

3 Rotation Extension
page 72

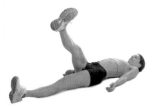

4 Wall Sit
page 94

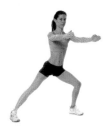

5 Lateral Low Lunge
page 82

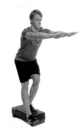

6 Step-Down
page 84

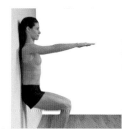

7 Unilateral Leg Circles
page 106

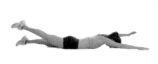

8 Swimming
page 110

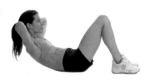

9 Basic Crunch
page 122

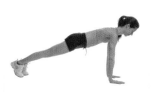

10 Push-Up
page 120

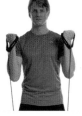

11 Biceps Curl
page 112

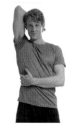

12 Triceps Extension
page 115

INTERMEDIATE STRENGTHENING WORKOUT

When you start feeling the results of your marathon training, try this series of exercises.

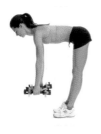

1 Dumbbell Deadlift
page 88

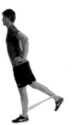

2 Hip Extension/Hip Flexion
page 76/page 77

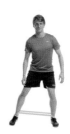

3 Side Steps
page 74

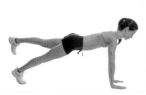

4 Plank Leg Extension
page 100

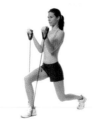

5 Resistance Band Lunge
page 90

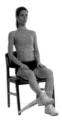

6 Rotation Extension
page 72

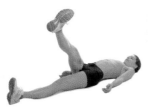

7 Unilateral Leg Circles
page 106

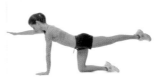

8 Quadruped Leg Lift
page 108

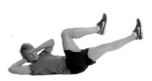

9 Crossover Crunch
page 124

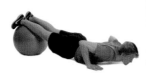

10 Swiss Ball Push-Up
page 132

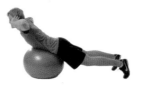

11 Swiss Ball Extension
page 136

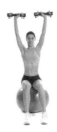

12 Swiss Ball Shoulder Press
page 114

ADVANCED STRENGTHENING WORKOUT

Challenge yourself with this targeted set of muscle strengtheners.

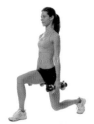

1 Dumbbell Lunge
page 92

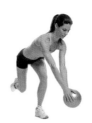

2 Power Squat
page 102

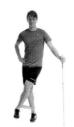

3 Hip Abduction and Adduction
page 73

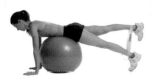

4 Swiss Ball Loop Extension
page 98

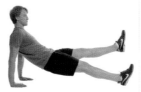

5 Front Plank Extension
page 140

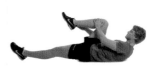

6 Abdominal Kick
page 126

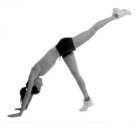

7 Three-Legged Dog
page 144

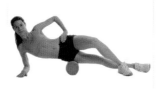

8 Iliotibial Band Release
page 130

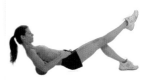

9 Roller Bridge with Leg Lift
page 142

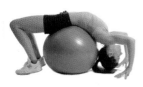

10 Backward Ball Stretch
page 138

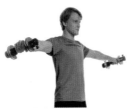

11 Lateral Shoulder Raise
page 116

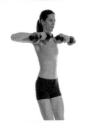

12 Frontal Raise and Row
page 118

CORE FOCUS FOR RUNNERS

A strong core is essential for a marathoner, so try this workout to enhance your training.

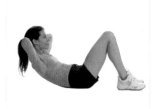

1 Basic Crunch
page 122

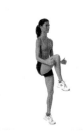

2 Standing Knee Crunch
page 128

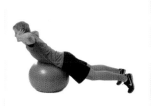

3 Swiss Ball Extension
page 136

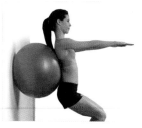

4 Swiss Ball Wall Squats
page 96

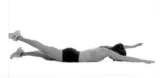

5 Swimming
page 110

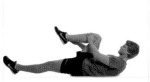

6 Abdominal Kick
page 126

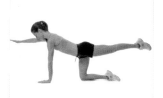

7 Quadruped Leg Lift
page 108

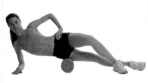

8 Iliotibial Band Release
page 130

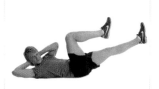

9 Crossover Crunch
page 124

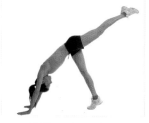

10 Three-Legged Dog
page 144

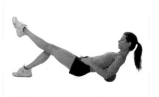

11 Roller Bridge with Leg Lift
page 142

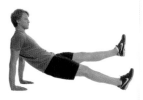

12 Front Plank Extension
page 140

RUNNERS' FULL-BODY WORKOUT

Here is a full-body workout that works both primary and secondary running muscles.

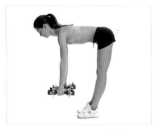

1 Dumbbell Deadlift
page 88

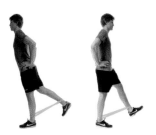

2 Hip Extension/Hip Flexion
page 76/page 77

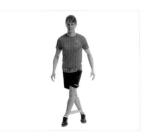

3 Crosssover Steps
page 75

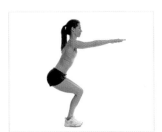

4 Knee Squat
page 80

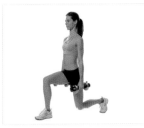

5 Dumbbell Lunge
page 92

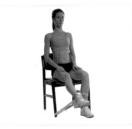

6 Rotation Extension
page 72

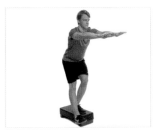

7 Step-Down
page 84

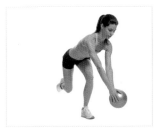

8 Power Squat
page 102

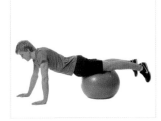

9 Swiss Ball Walkout
page 134

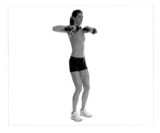

10 Frontal Raise and Row
page 118

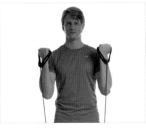

11 Biceps Curl
page 112

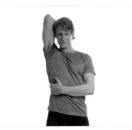

12 Triceps Extension
page 115

GLOSSARY

GENERAL TERMS

abduction: Movement away from the body.

adduction: Movement toward the body.

aerobic step: A portable step or platform with adjustable risers designed for cardiovascular exercising that also allows you to effectively work your calf muscles.

agonist muscle: See *antagonist muscle.*

anterior: Located in the front.

antagonist muscle: A muscle working in opposition to another, called the *agonist*. Most muscles work in antagonistic pairs, with one muscle contracting as the other expands; for example, when the biceps brachii contracts, the triceps brachii relaxes.

cardiovascular exercise: Any exercise that increases the heart rate, making oxygen and nutrient-rich blood available to muscles.

core: Refers to the deep muscle layers that lie close to the spine and provide structural support for the entire body. The core is divisible into two groups: the major core and the minor core. The major muscles reside on the trunk and include the belly area and the mid and lower back. This area encompasses the pelvic floor muscles (levator ani, pubococcygeus, iliococcygeus, puborectalis, and coccygeus), the abdominals (rectus abdominis, transversus abdominis, obliquus externus, and obliquus internus), the spinal extensors (multifidus spinae, erector spinae, splenius, longissimus thoracis, and semispinalis), and the diaphragm. The minor core muscles include the latissimus dorsi, gluteus maximus, and trapezius. Minor core muscles assist the major muscles when the body engages in activities or movements that require added stability.

crunch: A common abdominal exercise that calls for curling the shoulders toward the pelvis while lying supine with hands behind the head and knees bent.

curl: An exercise movement, usually targeting the biceps brachii, that calls for a weight to be moved through an arc, in a "curling" motion.

deadlift: An exercise movement that calls for lifting a weight, such as a dumbbell, off the floor from a stabilized bent-over position.

dumbbell: A basic piece of equipment that consists of a short bar on which plates are secured. A person can use a dumbbell in one or both hands during an exercise. Most gyms offer dumbbells with the weight plates welded on and poundage indicated on the plates, but many dumbbells intended for home use come with removable plates that allow you to adjust the weight.

extension: The act of straightening.

extensor muscle: A muscle serving to extend a body part away from the body.

flexion: The bending of a joint.

flexor muscle: A muscle that decreases the angle between two bones, as when bending the arm at the elbow or raising the thigh toward the stomach.

foam roller: A tube that comes in a variety of sizes, materials, and densities that can be used for stretching, strengthening, balance training, stability training, and self-massage.

gait cycle: The rhythmic alternating movements of the legs that result in the forward movement of the body, or the way we run or walk.

hamstrings: The three muscles of the posterior thigh (the semitendinosus, semimembranosus, and biceps femoris) that work to flex the knee and extend the hip.

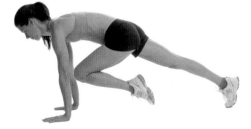

hand weight: Any of a range of free weights that are often used in weight training and toning. Small hand weights are usually cast iron formed in the shape of a dumbbell, sometimes coated with rubber or neoprene.

iliotibial band (ITB): A thick band of fibrous tissue that runs down the outside of the leg, beginning at the hip and extending to the outer side of the tibia just below the knee joint. The band functions in concert with several of the thigh muscles to provide stability to the outside of the knee joint.

lateral: Located on, or extending toward, the outside.

medial: Located on, or extending toward, the middle.

medicine ball: A small weighted ball used in weight training and toning.

neutral position (spine): A spinal position resembling an S shape, consisting of a inward curve in the lower back when viewed in profile.

posterior: Located behind.

press: An exercise movement that calls for moving a weight or other resistance away from the body.

primary muscle. One of the main muscles activated during a certain activity.

pronation. Turning inward. A pronated foot is one in which the heel bone angles inward and the arch tends to collapse. Opposite of *supination*.

quadriceps: A large muscle group (full name: quadriceps femoris) that includes the four prevailing muscles on the front of the thigh: the rectus femoris, vastus intermedius, vastus lateralis, and vastus medialis. It is the great extensor muscle of the knee, forming a large fleshy mass that covers the front and sides of the femur muscle.

range of motion: The distance and direction a joint can move between the flexed position and the extended position.

resistance band: Any rubber tubing or flat band device that provides a resistive force used for strength training. Also called a "fitness band," "Thera-Band," "Dyna-Band," "stretching band," and "exercise band."

rotator muscle: One of a group of muscles that assist the rotation of a joint, such as the hip or the shoulder.

scapula: The protrusion of bone on the mid to upper back, also known as the "shoulder blade."

secondary muscle: A muscle activated during a certain activity that usually works to support the primary muscles.

squat: An exercise movement that calls for moving the hips back and bending the knees and hips to lower the torso and an accompanying weight, and then returning to the upright position. A squat primarily targets the muscles of the thighs, hips, buttocks, and hamstrings.

supination: Turning outward. In running, supination is the insufficient inward roll of the foot after landing. This places extra stress on the foot and can result in iliotibial band syndrome, Achilles tendonitis, or plantar fasciitis. Also know as "overpronation."

Swiss ball: A flexile, inflatable PVC ball measuring approximately 18 to 30 inches (45 to 75 cm) in diameter that is used for weight training, physical therapy, balance training, and many other exercise regimens. It is also called a "balance ball," "fitness ball," "stability ball," "exercise ball," "gym ball," "physioball," "body ball," "therapy ball," and many other names.

warm-up: Any form of light exercise of short duration that prepares the body for more intense exercises.

weight: Refers to the plates or weight stacks, or the actual poundage listed on the bar or dumbbell.

LATIN TERMS

The following glossary explains the Latin scientific terminology used to describe the muscles of the human body. Certain words are derived from Greek, which is indicated in each instance.

CHEST

coracobrachialis: Greek *korakoeidés*, 'ravenlike,' and *brachium*, 'arm'

pectoralis (major and minor): *pectus*, 'breast'

ABDOMEN

obliquus externus: *obliquus*, 'slanting,' and *externus*, 'outward'

obliquus internus: *obliquus*, 'slanting,' and *internus*, 'within'

rectus abdominis: *rego*, 'straight, upright,' and *abdomen*, 'belly'

serratus anterior: *serra*, 'saw,' and *ante*, 'before'

transversus abdominis: *transversus*, 'athwart,' and *abdomen*, 'belly'

NECK

scalenus: Greek *skalénós*, 'unequal'

semispinalis: *semi*, 'half,' and *spinae*, 'spine'

splenius: Greek *spléníon*, 'plaster, patch'

sternocleidomastoideus: Greek *stérnon*, 'chest,' Greek *kleís*, 'key' and Greek *mastoeidés*, 'breastlike'

BACK

erector spinae: *erectus*, 'straight,' and *spina*, 'thorn'

latissimus dorsi: *latus*, 'wide,' and *dorsum*, 'back'

multifidus spinae: *multifid*, 'to cut into divisions,' and *spinae*, 'spine'

quadratus lumborum: *quadratus*, 'square, rectangular,' and *lumbus*, 'loin'

rhomboideus: Greek *rhembesthai*, 'to spin'

trapezius: Greek *trapezion*, 'small table'

SHOULDERS

deltoideus (anterior, medial, and posterior): Greek *deltoeidés*, 'delta-shaped'

infraspinatus: *infra*, 'under,' and *spina*, 'thorn'

levator scapulae: *levare*, 'to raise,' and *scapulae*, 'shoulder [blades]'

subscapularis: *sub*, 'below,' and *scapulae*, 'shoulder [blades]'

supraspinatus: *supra*, 'above,' and *spina*, 'thorn'

teres (major and minor): *teres*, 'rounded'

UPPER ARM

biceps brachii: *biceps*, 'two-headed,' and *brachium*, 'arm'

brachialis: *brachium*, 'arm'

triceps brachii: *triceps*, 'three-headed' and *brachium*, 'arm'

LOWER ARM

anconeus: Greek *anconad*, 'elbow'

brachioradialis: *brachium*, 'arm,' and *radius*, 'spoke'

extensor carpi radialis: *extendere*, 'to extend,' Greek *karpós*, 'wrist' and *radius*, 'spoke'

extensor digitorum: *extendere*, 'to extend,' and *digitus*, 'finger, toe'

flexor carpi pollicis longus: *flectere*, 'to bend,' Greek *karpós*, 'wrist,' *pollicis*, 'thumb' and *longus*, 'long'

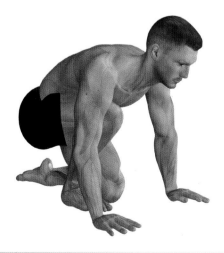

flexor carpi radialis: *flectere*, 'to bend,' Greek *karpós*, 'wrist' and *radius*, 'spoke'

flexor carpi ulnaris: *flectere*, 'to bend,' Greek *karpós*, 'wrist,' and *ulnaris*, 'forearm'

flexor digitorum: *flectere*, 'to bend,' and *digitus*, 'finger, toe'

palmaris longus: *palmaris*, 'palm,' and *longus*, 'long'

pronator teres: *pronate*, 'to rotate,' and *teres*, 'rounded'

HIPS

gemellus (inferior and superior): *geminus*, 'twin'

gluteus maximus: Greek *gloutós*, 'rump,' and *maximus*, 'largest'

gluteus medius: Greek *gloutós*, 'rump' and *medialis*, 'middle'

gluteus minimus: Greek *gloutós*, 'rump' and *minimus*, 'smallest'

iliopsoas: *ilium*, 'groin,' and Greek *psoa*, 'groin muscle'

obturator externus: *obturare*, 'to block' and *externus*, 'outward'

obturator internus: *obturare*, 'to block' and *internus*, 'within'

pectineus: *pectin*, 'comb'

piriformis: *pirum*, 'pear,' and *forma*, 'shape'

quadratus femoris: *quadratus*, 'square, rectangular,' and *femur*, 'thigh'

UPPER LEG

adductor longus: *adducere*, 'to contract,' and *longus*, 'long'

adductor magnus: *adducere*, 'to contract,' and *magnus*, 'major'

biceps femoris: *biceps*, 'two-headed,' and *femur*, 'thigh'

gracilis: *gracilis*, 'slim, slender'

rectus femoris: *rego*, 'straight, upright,' and *femur*, 'thigh'

sartorius: *sarcio*, 'to patch' or 'to repair'

semimembranosus: *semi*, 'half,' and *membrum*, 'limb'

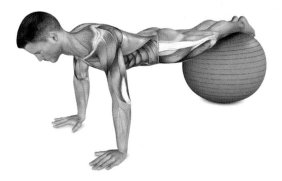

semitendinosus: *semi*, 'half,' and *tendo*, 'tendon'

tensor fasciae latae: *tenere*, 'to stretch,' *fasciae*, 'band,' and *latae*, 'laid down'

vastus intermedius: *vastus*, 'immense, huge,' and *intermedius*, 'between'

vastus lateralis: *vastus*, 'immense, huge,' and *lateralis*, 'side'

vastus medialis: *vastus*, 'immense, huge,' and *medialis*, 'middle'

LOWER LEG

adductor digiti minimi: *adducere*, 'to contract,' *digitus*, 'finger, toe,' and *minimum* 'smallest'

adductor hallucis: *adducere*, 'to contract,' and *hallex*, 'big toe'

extensor digitorum longus: *extendere*, 'to extend,' *digitus*, 'finger, toe' and *longus*, 'long'

extensor hallucis longus: *extendere*, 'to extend,' *hallex*, 'big toe,' and *longus*, 'long'

flexor digitorum longus: *flectere*, 'to bend,' *digitus*, 'finger, toe' and *longus*, 'long'

flexor hallucis longus: *flectere*, 'to bend,' and *hallex*, 'big toe' and *longus*, 'long'

gastrocnemius: Greek *gastroknémía*, 'calf [of the leg]'

peroneus: *peronei*, 'of the fibula'

plantaris: *planta*, 'the sole'

soleus: *solea*, 'sandal'

tibialis anterior: *tibia*, 'reed pipe,' and *ante*, 'before'

tibialis posterior: *tibia*, 'reed pipe,' and *posterus*, 'coming after'

CREDITS

Created by Lisa Purcell Editorial & Design for Moseley Road Inc.

Moseley Road Inc.
123 Main Street
Irvington, New York 10533

President: Sean Moore
Production director: Adam Moore
Project art and editorial director: Lisa Purcell

Photographer: Jonathan Conklin Photography, Inc.

Models: Sara Blowers and Nicolay Alexandrov

Illustrator: Hector Aiza/3D Labz Animation India (www.3dlabz.com)

All photographs by Jonathan Conklin except the following: background image by fotomak/Shutterstock.com; 8 ostill/Shutterstock.com; 11, 22 bottom Warren Goldswain/Shutterstock.com; 12, 13 right, 14, 15, 19, 20 left Maridav/Shutterstock.com; 13 left arka38/Shutterstock.com; 16 Suzanne Tucker/Shutterstock.com; 18 PeterG/Shutterstock.com; 21 Marc Dietrich/Shutterstock.com; 23 Monkey Business Images/Shutterstock.com; 24 left Richard Waters/Shutterstock.com.

All illustrations by Hector Aiza except the following: Insets and page 24 right, 25 design36/Shutterstock.com; 20 right, 22 top Alila Medical Media/Shutterstock.com; 26, 27 Linda Bucklin/Shutterstock.com

ABOUT THE AUTHORS

Dr. Philip Striano is the owner of Hudson Rivertown's Chiropractic Health Care in Dobbs Ferry, New York. He is a certified chiropractic sports physician and a sports injury, exercise, and strength and conditioning specialist. He received his doctor of chiropractic degree from New York Chiropractic College.

Lisa Purcell is a New York City book designer, editor, and writer. A graduate of Princeton University, she specializes in health and fitness books.